P9-AER-623

Resounding praise for
ESTROGEN MATTERS

"How could one flawed scientific conclusion become a persuasive juggernaut that changed the practice of women's health worldwide? In their fascinating account, Bluming and Tavris challenge that conclusion and unpack the reasons for its remarkable impact."
—Robert B. Cialdini, PhD, author of *Influence* and *Pre-Suasion*

"This is such an important book, I want to do all I can to encourage every woman to read it. Groundbreaking and carefully researched, *Estrogen Matters* provides essential information about the many benefits of estrogen at menopause and even after a diagnosis of breast cancer. It reveals the misinterpretation of study results that led women (and their doctors) to have unwarranted concerns about estrogen use. The thoughtful information presented here will help women feel more comfortable taking estrogen, leading to healthier, longer lives for many."
—Patricia T. Kelly, PhD, specialist in cancer risk assessment and author of *Assessing Your True Risk of Breast Cancer*

"Given breast cancer's substantial morbidity, mortality, emotional toll, and the vast consequences of its treatment, this frontal salvo on the conventional wisdom of estrogen use is refreshing and welcome. The book will stir a lively debate about the merits of decades of existing clinical research on estrogens and help reframe the way clinicians and patients view the trade-off between the benefits and risks of hormone therapy."
—Jerome P. Kassirer, MD, distinguished professor, Tufts University School of Medicine, and former editor in chief, *New England Journal of Medicine*

"Having spent over two decades advancing women's health, I was appalled by the Women's Health Initiative's efforts to sensationalize and distort their own findings to promote an anti-hormone-therapy agenda. I hope *Estrogen Matters* draws enough attention to counter the fears and misinformation about HRT that so many women, and their physicians, still hold."

—Phyllis Greenberger, MSW, former president and CEO of the Society for Women's Health Research

"This book is long overdue, and I salute the authors for their courage and effort (and their clear, witty writing). I believe it is an ethical imperative for all clinicians who treat women in menopause or women with breast cancer to alert their patients to this book."

—Michael Baum, MD, Visiting Professor of Medical Humanities, University College London

"Bluming and Tavris tell estrogen's story in a way that is both accessible to the general public and appropriate for professionals. This book is an exhaustively researched and meticulously reasoned vindication of HRT. Very enlightening!"

—Harriet Hall, MD, editor, *Science-Based Medicine*

"Well-written, insightful, and hard-hitting, *Estrogen Matters* successfully rebuts the billion-dollar government-led study known as the Women's Health Initiative, which claimed that hormones for postmenopausal women are harmful. That study was wrong. It turns out estrogens do matter for women's health."

—Vincent T. DeVita Jr., MD, professor of medicine, Yale Cancer Center, and professor of epidemiology and public health, Yale Medical School

Estrogen Matters

Why Taking Hormones in Menopause
Can Improve Women's Well-Being and
Lengthen Their Lives—Without Raising
the Risk of Breast Cancer

Avrum Bluming, MD,
and Carol Tavris, PhD

Little, Brown Spark
New York Boston London

This book is intended to provide helpful and informative material, including the opinions and conclusions of the authors with respect to some vitally important yet controversial medical issues. It is not intended to replace the advice of a physician. Always consult your physician or qualified health-care professional on any matters regarding your health and before adopting any suggestions in this book or drawing inferences from it.

The author and publisher specifically disclaim any liability, loss, or risk, personal or otherwise, that is incurred as a consequence, directly or indirectly, of the use and application of any of the contents of this book.

Copyright © 2018 by Avrum Bluming, MD, and Carol Tavris, PhD
Afterword 2021 copyright © 2021 by Avrum Bluming, MD, and Carol Tavris, PhD

Hachette Book Group supports the right to free expression and the value of copyright. The purpose of copyright is to encourage writers and artists to produce the creative works that enrich our culture.

The scanning, uploading, and distribution of this book without permission is a theft of the author's intellectual property. If you would like permission to use material from the book (other than for review purposes), please contact permissions@hbgusa.com. Thank you for your support of the author's rights.

Little, Brown Spark
Hachette Book Group
1290 Avenue of the Americas, New York, NY 10104
littlebrownspark.com

First Edition: September 2018

Little, Brown Spark is an imprint of Little, Brown and Company, a division of Hachette Book Group, Inc. The Little, Brown Spark name and logo are trademarks of Hachette Book Group, Inc.

The publisher is not responsible for websites (or their content) that are not owned by the publisher.

The Hachette Speakers Bureau provides a wide range of authors for speaking events. To find out more, go to hachettespeakersbureau.com or call (866) 376-6591.

ISBN 978-0-316-48120-5
LCCN 2018939458

Printing 7, 2022

LSC-C

Printed in the United States of America

To my patients, whose trust, courage, understanding, and
cooperation made my research possible,
and to my wife, Martha, who makes anything possible.
—Avrum Bluming

Contents

Introduction: Who Killed HRT?   3

1. Does Estrogen Cause Breast Cancer?   17
2. The "Change of Life" and the Quality of Life   55
3. Matters of the Heart   83
4. Breaking Bad   105
5. Losing and Using Our Minds   127
6. Can Breast Cancer Survivors Take Estrogen?   163
7. Progesterone and the Pill   195
8. Debates, Decisions, and Final Lessons in the
   Case for HRT   211
   Afterword   241

Acknowledgments   244
Notes   247
Index   303

Facts will ultimately preempt statistics.

— Bernadine Healy

Truth is the daughter of time, not of authority.

— Francis Bacon

Estrogen
Matters

Introduction

Who Killed HRT?

Avrum recently received an e-mail from a woman he did not know, referred to him by a mutual friend, who was agonizing over suspicious findings on her breast ultrasound. Her mammogram had shown a probable cyst, so the radiologist had ordered the ultrasound, and the results suggested a malignancy. The woman wrote that she was "freaking out," feeling hopeless, and already anticipating a total mastectomy; she added that if she could have her whole torso surgically removed, she would. This woman was a fifty-year-old university professor of experimental psychology, yet she was completely panicked before a biopsy had even been performed.

Av is profoundly aware of the fear that accompanies even a suspicion of a breast cancer diagnosis. He has been a medical oncologist for many years, and about 60 percent of his practice has been devoted to the study and treatment of breast cancer. In 1988, his wife, Martha, was diagnosed with breast cancer at the age of forty-five. She had found a small nodule that seemed benign but nonetheless warranted removal, and he vividly remembers his own fear when the surgeon who removed the tumor said, "I'm sorry, Av. It was a carcinoma." He felt as though he had been walking along a rocky path on a high mountain, holding Martha's hand, and they had suddenly lost their footing. Two days later, the surgeon told them almost casually that the nodes he'd sent for biopsy when he removed the tumor appeared completely normal. Av regained his balance. Whatever else might turn up, there was now a good chance that Martha would be cured.

The often repeated statistic that one woman in eight (12 percent) will develop breast cancer at some point in her life should be understood in a broader context: That's a woman's risk of getting it, all right, but only if she lives to be eighty-five. As Patricia T. Kelly explained in *Assess Your True Risk of Breast Cancer:*

- A thirty-year-old woman has a risk of developing breast cancer *in the next decade* of 1 in 227 (0.4 percent).
- A forty-year-old woman has a decade risk of 1 in 68 (1.5 percent).
- A fifty-year-old woman has a decade risk of 1 in 42 (2.4 percent).
- A sixty-year-old woman has a decade risk of 1 in 28 (3.6 percent).
- A woman over seventy has the highest risk, 1 in 26 (4 percent).[1]

So where did that one-in-eight risk come from? It's obtained by adding together the risks in each age category: 0.4 plus 1.5 plus 2.4

and so forth. But if you are a woman who has reached age sixty without a diagnosis of breast cancer, your risk in the coming decades is only 7.6 percent (12 percent less each decade's risk that you have passed); the risk of breast cancer in any given decade of life never exceeds one in *twenty-six.* Yet by far the most important statistic is this one: over 90 percent of women currently diagnosed with early breast cancer will be cured, and most will not need disfiguring mastectomies or chemotherapy.

Martha's cancer was diagnosed thirty years ago. After her lumpectomy, she received postoperative radiotherapy and chemotherapy and has had no recurrence of cancer since. The chemotherapy she received, however, pushed her into menopause; severe symptoms began and then continued unabated. She didn't complain, understanding better than her husband did what women were expected to tolerate at that time as part of the "change of life." But she was most definitely suffering. For years, the women under Av's care had been reporting a variety of the same symptoms: hot flashes, loss of sexual desire, painful intercourse because of vaginal dryness, difficulty sleeping, palpitations, unexplained and uncharacteristic anxiety attacks, difficulty concentrating, and — the thing that especially bothered Martha — fuzzy thinking, such as trouble remembering phone numbers and even following the plot of a book.

And so Avrum delved more systematically into the world of menopausal symptoms and their treatments. At the time, and still today, the uncontested most effective treatment for these symptoms was — and is — estrogen. Because estrogen replacement therapy (ERT) alone is associated with an increased risk of endometrial cancer (cancer of the lining of the uterus), women who still have a uterus are given hormone replacement therapy (HRT)—estrogen plus progesterone—which provides the benefits of estrogen without the increased risk of endometrial cancer.* Martha asked Av about prescribing estrogen for her. Many of his menopausal patients who had been treated for breast cancer over the years had asked for the same thing. They had complained of severe quality-of-life impairments that they hoped estrogen would alleviate. He had advised against it because of the prevalent concern that estrogen might increase the risk of cancer recurrence among women with previous breast cancer. (As you will learn in chapter 6, it does not.)

By the early 1990s, researchers had fifty years of evidence of estrogen's benefits, all of it well documented in the medical literature. Estrogen not only successfully controlled menopausal symptoms in most women but also significantly reduced the risks of heart disease, hip fractures, colon cancer, and Alzheimer's. A 1991 *New England Journal of Medicine* editorial, "Uncertainty About Postmenopausal Estrogen: Time for Action, Not Debate," reported a 40 to 50 percent reduction in atherosclerotic heart disease, which was responsible for the deaths of more than eight times as many American women as breast cancer.[2] The long-running Framingham study reported a 50 percent drop in osteoporosis-associated hip fractures, which were linked to as many deaths every year as breast cancer.[3] Two studies, one from the University of Wisconsin

---

* These acronyms are currently under debate because many physicians and laypeople dislike the word *replacement*. Some prefer *hormone therapy* (although that term could refer to taking any hormones for any problem), and others like *menopausal hormone therapy*, which doesn't seem to be much of an improvement. Because ERT and HRT are still in common use and clearly distinguish estrogen therapy alone from therapy with combined hormones, those are the terms we will use in this book.

and one from the American Cancer Society, reported a 50 percent decrease in the risk of developing or dying of colon cancer. And a USC study reported a 35 percent decrease in the risk of Alzheimer's. Among women with no history of breast cancer, studies found that estrogen did not increase the risk of developing it, even among women who had been taking estrogen for ten to fifteen years. Most remarkable, women taking estrogen were living longer than women who were not taking hormones. A 1997 report in the *Journal of the American Medical Association* stated that "HRT should increase life expectancy for nearly all postmenopausal women by up to 3 years."[4] Their analysis concluded that up to 99 percent of current postmenopausal women would benefit from taking HRT as measured by decreased rates of disease and improved longevity.

So it is no wonder that in the 1990s, the medical consensus was fairly strong about the benefits of ERT and HRT. In her 1995 book *A New Prescription for Women's Health: Getting the Best Medical Care in a Man's World*, Bernadine Healy, a cardiologist and the first (and thus far only) female director of the National Institutes of Health (NIH), observed that many of the major risks that women face as they age—heart disease, stroke, osteoporosis, and Alzheimer's disease—"are or may well be reduced by hormone replacement therapy." As a result of that data, she wrote, when she hit menopause, she planned to begin HRT "without a blink":

> To me, the benefits are nothing short of remarkable. Distilling all the reports, I conclude that long-term hormone replacement therapy may not make one feminine forever, but it clearly offers the chance for being healthier far longer. The benefits of hormone replacement therapy on individual

diseases or specific organs are impressive. But when the benefits are looked at in aggregate, they are compelling. The total health of a woman as she gets older is largely what determines her quality of life, what allows her to view the last half of her adult life as a blessing and a second prime.[5]

And then she added: "A decision not to consider hormone replacement is a health decision, too, just as is the decision not to take a flu shot or get a hepatitis vaccination. As I see it, women have a competitive health and survival edge before menopause. Women during their childbearing years are protected against many problems that affect men. I see no reason to relinquish that advantage after menopause—not if I can help it."

Today, more than twenty years after Bernadine Healy's published advice, estrogen's benefits have been drowned out by the alarms about its risks, which were inflamed by reports from the Women's Health Initiative (WHI), initially published in 2002. Those reports claimed that HRT was flat-out dangerous, that it increased the risks of breast cancer, heart disease, stroke, and dementia, all leading to a shortened life expectancy. Hundreds of thousands of women, already frightened of breast cancer, went off hormone replacement immediately. Most of their physicians supported them. If you go online, you'll see how many establishment medical centers to this day rely on the WHI and advise women not to take HRT at all or to take it only briefly.

Yet, as we will show in a close examination of the WHI studies, some of those claims were exaggerated, some were misleading, and some were just wrong—and several WHI investigators themselves eventually backed away from them. We realize what a stunning assertion this is. The Women's Health Initiative, supposedly the gold standard of empirical research, funded by the National Institutes of Health to the tune of one billion dollars—and we are arguing that its findings can't be trusted? Yes, we are, and we hope that by the time you finish this book, you will see why.

While we're at it, we plan to shatter a widespread assumption underlying the concerns about HRT: that estrogen causes breast cancer. As Av began to question the received wisdom on estrogen, he found himself in the same position as the physicians who dared question the once universal belief in the benefits of radical mastectomy, promoted by the surgeon William Halsted in the late nineteenth and early twentieth centuries. Radical mastectomy was based in part on Halsted's theory that breast cancer spread almost exclusively from the original site into contiguous areas. Find a tumor in the breast? Then it is essential to remove the tumor, the entire breast, and everything adjacent—a "radical" procedure.

Halsted's assumption was logical, widely accepted, and wrong. In the fifty-four years between 1927 and 1981, twenty-four studies reported on more than four thousand patients with breast cancer who were treated with lumpectomy (removal of the tumor only) and, usually, subsequent radiation. In all but two of those studies, survival rates, even up to thirty years later, were similar to those of patients treated with variations of the radical mastectomy. Randomized trials and observational studies continue to show that breast-conserving surgery is almost always at least as effective as mastectomy. Yet rates of radical mastectomies, especially bilateral mastectomies, for treatment of localized breast cancer have been rising since 2006—another manifestation of the fear associated with breast cancer. In the overwhelming majority of these cases, mastectomy is not indicated and not recommended. Yet many patients, like the woman who wrote to Avrum, panic and say, "Just take it off—take them both off—so I don't have to worry." They would rather cope with the pain, discomfort, prolonged recovery, and physical impairments of extensive surgery than deal with anxiety, even though the more extensive surgery does not offer a greater chance for cure.

Like Halsted's mistaken notion that breast cancer spreads from the original site to adjacent areas, the belief that estrogen causes breast cancer is logical, widely accepted, and wrong. Consider these findings, which you will learn more about in detail in this book:

- If estrogen were an important cause of breast cancer, we would expect rates of breast cancer to decline after menopause, when estrogen levels naturally diminish. Instead, breast cancer rates increase.
- If estrogen were carcinogenic, we would hardly expect it to be beneficial to women with breast cancer. You would not treat patients with lung cancer by dramatically increasing the number of cigarettes they smoke daily. But high doses of estrogen have been effectively used to treat metastatic breast cancer, and women diagnosed with breast cancer while on HRT or ERT have repeatedly been found to have a better prognosis than those diagnosed who are not taking it.
- The belief that a woman's lifetime, cumulative level of estrogen is a major contributor to breast cancer is based on weak and largely circumstantial evidence. It came from the perception that women who enter menarche very early (when estrogen levels start to rise) and have late menopause (when

estrogen declines sharply) have a higher risk of breast cancer. But they don't. Moreover, the endometrium (the lining of the uterus) is more sensitive to any tumor-promoting effects of estrogen than the breast. If "excess" estrogen were a mechanism by which age at menarche and age at menopause increased the risk of breast cancer, then the risk of endometrial cancer should also be related to these events. It is not.

- Some normal breast cells have on their cell membranes receptor molecules for estrogen, and many women diagnosed with estrogen-receptor-positive breast cancer assume, understandably, that this means that estrogen is somehow feeding the kind of breast cancer they have. But no. If that receptor is found on the membrane of a breast cancer cell, it usually means the breast cancer is growing slowly enough to adopt this normal cell characteristic. Indeed, in most breast cancers, estrogen-receptor-positive cells are *not* the ones proliferating. A similar receptor has been identified for progesterone. The presence of an estrogen receptor or a progesterone receptor on the surface of a breast cancer cell does not mean that the breast cancer was *caused* by estrogen or progesterone. Moreover, the cells of early breast cancer and the ones that multiply within breast cancer are generally estrogen-receptor and progesterone-receptor negative.[6]

- During pregnancy, circulating estrogen concentrations are at least ten times higher than during other periods of a woman's life. Yet women who are diagnosed with breast cancer during pregnancy have a similar prognosis as nonpregnant women at the same stages of breast cancer. Moreover, terminating the pregnancies in women with recently diagnosed breast cancer, thereby eliminating the increased level of circulating estrogen, produces no benefit for either its course or prognosis.

*   *   *

We—Avrum and Carol—have been close friends for many years. We met when Avrum saved Carol's sister-in-law's life with a successful intervention for a rare blood disorder caused by a stroke medication. We discovered a mutual passion for following the data wherever it led and a shared commitment to debunking pseudoscience and fad therapies, Av in medicine, Carol in psychology. The story of HRT, a therapy designed to treat life changes that are specific to women—a therapy praised by some researchers, condemned by others, and eventually brought down by a large nationwide study—was fascinating in its own right but was also a perfect case study for Carol's interest in gender biases in health care and cognitive biases in research.

And so, one afternoon more than a decade ago, Carol decided to attend Avrum's talk about HRT at a continuing-medical-education seminar. She went mostly out of friendship. She was not an advocate of hormones, nor did she have a vested interest in them one way or the other; she had sailed through menopause with nary a symptom. In her 1992 book *The Mismeasure of Woman,* she included a chapter on hormone replacement, a therapy she didn't wholly oppose but didn't wholly endorse either. In those years, she shared the view of many women's health activists that the idea of hormone "replacement" was itself problematic, implying that the normal changes of life automatically created deficiencies rather than being, well, normal changes of life.

And then she watched, riveted, as Avrum set about methodically dismantling the arguments stating that HRT was a serious risk factor in breast cancer. He presented a table of breast cancer risks (which you will see in chapter 1). At the lower end was taking Premarin—an insignificant risk. Riskier factors included eating fish, eating one additional serving of French fries per week during preschool years, and being a Scandinavian airline flight attendant. All of these associations were weak, unlikely, and meaningless in real life, and all were stronger than those with Premarin, but all of them found homes in medical journals.

Bingo! Carol realized that Avrum was doing in medicine what she loved doing in psychology: dealing with evidence that contradicted received wisdom and coming face-to-face with the exasperating reaction that most people have to such evidence. (They rarely say, "Thank you." They don't say much of anything.) She was therefore not surprised when Av told her how much trouble he was having in trying to persuade his colleagues that they might be wrong about the dangers of HRT and the reliability of the Women's Health Initiative. Carol offered to collaborate with him on articles for his medical colleagues, and these were soon published by the *Cancer Journal* and *Climacteric*.[7] The papers' detailed examinations of the disgraceful data manipulations of the WHI were greeted by the medical establishment with...silence.

And so, this book. Just as decades of evidence eventually overturned the scientific justification for radical mastectomy, decades of evidence indicates that it is time to change medical professionals' minds about estrogen too. We will show how the powerful belief that estrogen causes breast cancer has blinded otherwise reputable, serious investigators to what their own data actually reveals. And we will show how the powerful belief that advocates for estrogen are all in the pocket of Big Pharma—as, indeed, some of them are—has blinded many conscientious feminists, scientists, and health activists and kept them from taking that data seriously.

Accordingly, before we go any further, we want to make it clear that neither of us is a partially or wholly owned subsidiary of Wyeth (purchased by Pfizer in 2009) or any other drug company. Carol has long been an outspoken critic of the pharmaceutical industry, and Avrum does not and has not met with drug reps in his office, let alone accepted dinners, pens, speaking offers, writing assignments, pizzas, or any other bribe or inducement, in exchange for a prescription. In 2005, Avrum was contacted by a lawyer representing Wyeth, and he agreed to serve as an expert witness on a case, since his *already published* papers had questioned the role of hormones in the development of breast cancer. He was not hired to create an opinion.

Last year, Avrum got an e-mail from a former patient who had moved to another city.

Dear Dr. Bluming:

Today I had an appointment with Dr. L to renew my prescription for the hormones I have been taking. She quickly told me to find another doctor as she could not and would not prescribe HRT. In order for someone to be given hormones, she said, the patient would have to be no older than 62 or so (I am much older) and have hot flashes—which I do not have because I am on hormones. She would not continue to treat me if I insisted on remaining on hormones. She finally wrote a prescription for only one month and told me to go look for another doctor. These medicines have helped me a great deal and provided me with a life, instead of days of sitting on the sofa or in bed unable to move or think. What do I do? Who can I see? Are there other drugs I can take in their place? How can I find a doctor to support me and track what is needed?

As he read his patient's letter, Av wondered how her otherwise competent young oncologist had become so adamantly opposed to hormone replacement therapy that she was unable to recognize its benefits in the patient sitting in front of her, a woman who had been on HRT for more than twenty years. To answer that question, we will consider the effects of hormone replacement therapy on menopausal symptoms, heart disease, bone health, overall survival, and cancer and conclude with recommendations of where we go from here. If a woman is trying to choose whether or not to take ERT or HRT, she owes herself a familiarity with its benefits and risks, and that is what this book is designed to provide.

Every action that human beings take involves risk: crossing the street, swallowing an aspirin, getting married. In the case of estrogen, yes, of course, there are some legitimate concerns about risks, and we will discuss them. But we will argue that medical professionals, in their concern about what turn out to be small risks for *some* women, are overlooking the overwhelming evidence of estrogen's very large benefits for *most* women. Women have been scared away from estrogen by the fear of breast cancer—a fear so great that it made an educated woman like Avrum's correspondent claim she would sacrifice her "whole torso" for a cure, even before she had an official diagnosis of cancer. We hope this book will replace that fear with a deeper understanding that will allow women, with guidance from informed physicians, to make decisions based on knowledge rather than on unfounded anxiety and false alarms.

1

Does Estrogen Cause Breast Cancer?

Yes, it does." "No, it doesn't." Conjectures and controversies have swirled around this question for more than a hundred years, and that fact alone provides a clue to the answer. The Nobel Prize–winning physicist Richard Feynman had a good test for truth in science: "If something is true, really so," he said, "if you continue observations and improve the effectiveness of the observations, the effects stand out more obviously."[1] If you continue your observations and all you get are muddy and inconsistent answers, something is wrong with your method or, more likely, with your hypothesis.

Advances in science are rarely achieved by one dramatic insight or experimental finding. They are usually the result of small steps and conclusions, many of which point in the same general direction, allowing the evolution of an idea that can then be tested and either verified or disproved. Unfortunately, not all scientists are as dispassionate in their pursuit of a finding as Feynman was. For him, being wrong was as informative as being right. But many scientists, like almost all mortals, would rather be right—and some, as we will see in this chapter, are willing to bend their experiments' findings to fit their theories.

Efforts to understand and treat breast cancer have a long history.[2] In the late 1800s, a few physicians suggested there might be a causal relationship between a product of the ovary, most likely estrogen, and the development and progression of breast cancer. In 1882, Thomas William Nunn reported the case history of a perimenopausal woman with breast cancer whose disease regressed six months after her periods stopped. In 1889, Albert Schinzinger, observing that breast cancer was less aggressive in older women than in younger women, proposed that removing both ovaries in premenopausal women with breast cancer would send them into early menopause and thus cause the breast cancer to regress. Schinzinger never performed the surgery, however, because he was unable to convince his colleagues of its potential merit. But six years later, in 1895, George Thomas Beatson removed both ovaries of a woman who had extensive, recurrent breast cancer. The patient's tumor regressed completely and she survived for four years after the surgery. One year later, in 1896, Stanley Boyd, an English surgeon, removed both ovaries in a woman with metastatic breast cancer; she survived for twelve years after her surgery. Boyd later wrote, "My working hypothesis is that internal secretion of the ovaries in some cases favors the growth of the cancer."

There matters stood for almost half a century.

In 1942, researchers developed methods to extract large quantities of estrogen from the urine of pregnant mares, and Ayerst Laboratories produced the first estrogen tablets, which they called Premarin (from *preg*nant *mare*'s ur*ine*). Ayerst began to market Premarin in the 1950s as a treatment for menopausal symptoms, a campaign greatly enhanced in the 1960s by the publication of *Feminine Forever*, a hyperventilating bestseller written by New York gynecologist Robert Wilson.[3] The book promised youth, beauty, and a full sex life for menopausal women through the use of estrogen. Wilson's son Ronald later told reporter Gina Kolata at the *New York Times* that Ayerst had paid all of his father's expenses for writing the book and financed his father's organization, the Wilson Research Foundation.[4]

This euphoric endorsement of estrogen was tempered by the discovery in the 1970s that the incidence of endometrial cancer, a generally curable cancer of the cells lining the uterus, was increased four to eight times in all those "feminine forever" women taking estrogen.[5] Subsequent studies reported that the addition of progesterone, another female hormone, not only negated the increased risk of uterine cancer associated with estrogen alone but actually protected against endometrial cancer; women receiving progesterone with estrogen had a lower incidence of endometrial cancer than women who received no hormones.[6] That is why, ever since the early 1980s, women who have had hysterectomies and who subsequently start hormone therapy get estrogen alone (ERT), while women who have not undergone hysterectomies and who start hormone therapy receive estrogen plus progesterone (HRT). Varieties of synthetic progesterone, developed to improve the absorption of the drug, are referred to as progestins.

Today, the major concern among physicians, women's health

activists, and laypeople is not uterine cancer but breast cancer—and the possible role of hormones in causing it. Throughout the 1980s and 1990s, however, there was little evidence to warrant that concern. On the contrary, there was a drumbeat of reassuring findings:

- A 1986 study led by epidemiologist Louise Brinton at the National Cancer Institute found no statistically significant increased risk of breast cancer among women on Premarin, even among those who had been taking it for more than twenty years.[7]

- A 1988 meta-analysis of twenty-two studies by Bruce Armstrong at the Research Unit in Epidemiology and Preventive Medicine of the University of Western Australia found no statistical association between ERT and breast cancer.[8]

- A 1991 study led by epidemiologist Julie Palmer at Boston University School of Medicine found no increased risk of breast cancer among Premarin users even after fifteen years of use.[9]

- A 1991 analysis of twenty-eight studies by biostatistician William Dupont and pathologist David L. Page at the Vanderbilt University School of Medicine found no association between ERT and breast cancer.[10]

- In 1992, the first randomized, double-blind, placebo-controlled trial on this subject was published. Twenty-two years earlier, obstetrician-gynecologist and medical researcher Lila Nachtigall and her colleagues at New York University Langone Medical Center had randomly assigned 168 postmenopausal women who were continuously hospitalized in a mental institution to receive either HRT or placebo. After more than two decades, 11.5 percent of the women taking the placebo had developed breast cancer—but *none* of the women on HRT had.[11]

- Because women who undergo biopsies for benign breast disease have a slight increased risk of breast cancer, researchers followed 3,303 women who had benign breast biopsies performed at Vanderbilt University between 1958 and 1960. The median duration of the follow-up was seventeen years. In this study, published in 1989, women who were given estrogen following the biopsy—even those who had a family history of breast cancer—did not subsequently have an increased risk of breast cancer themselves.[12]

Of course there were a few contradictory studies—there always are in medicine—but by the year 2000, major journals, research institutions, and leading oncologists were coming to the consensus that estrogen did not increase the risk of breast cancer.

A 1987 consensus development conference, reported in the *British Medical Journal* (*BMJ*), concluded that "well-defined epidemiological studies of ERT do not suggest an overall increase in the risk of breast cancer in postmenopausal women."[13]

In a 1993 editorial in the *New England Journal of Medicine* (*NEJM*), endocrinologists Kathryn Martin and Mason Freeman of Massachusetts General Hospital, Harvard, stated, "On the basis of the available evidence, we recommend that all postmenopausal women be considered candidates for hormone replacement therapy and be educated about its risks and benefits."[14]

According to a 1995 study by epidemiologist Janet Stanford of the University of Washington, "The use of estrogen with progestin (HRT) does not appear to be associated with an increased risk of breast cancer.... Compared with nonusers of menopausal hormones, those who used estrogen-progestin HRT for eight or more years had, if anything, a reduced risk of breast cancer."[15]

A 1995 article in the *New England Journal of Medicine* reported the first wave of results from the Nurses' Health Study, which involved 121,700 female registered nurses who were followed from 1976 through 1992. The women who had used HRT at any point, even those who had been taking it for more than ten years, had no increased risk of breast cancer compared to women who never took HRT.[16]

A 1996 prospective study of 422,373 women, led by Dawn Willis and conducted under the auspices of the American Cancer Society, found that those who had ever taken estrogen replacement therapy had a small but significantly decreased risk of dying of breast cancer.[17]

A 1997 article by Nananda Col, a researcher then at the New England Medical Center and the Tufts University School of Medicine, concluded: "Our analysis suggests that HRT will result in gains in life expectancy for most newly postmenopausal women and that these gains may exceed 3 years in some women."[18]

In 1997, epidemiologist Thomas Sellers at the Moffitt Cancer Center of the University of Minnesota studied a random sample of 41,837 female Iowa residents between fifty-five and sixty-nine years of age to determine whether HRT was associated with an increased risk of breast cancer in women with a family history of breast cancer. It was not.[19]

In 2006, biostatistician Masahiro Takeuchi, at the National Cancer Center Hospital in Tokyo, studied nine thousand Japanese women and found that those who were on HRT were less likely to develop breast cancer than never-users.[20]

In 2006, the Women's Health Initiative—about which we will have much more to say—reported no increased risk of breast cancer in postmenopausal women who had been on ERT, even after seven years of follow-up.[21]

In 2005, a stunning and counterintuitive discovery was made by the epidemiologist Timothy Rebbeck and his colleagues at the University of Pennsylvania School of Medicine. They studied 462 pre- and postmenopausal women with the BRCA1 and BRCA2 mutations, which are known to increase the risk of ovarian and of breast cancer. BRCA-positive women are usually advised to have both ovaries removed because that procedure dramatically reduces the risk of ovarian cancer and cuts the subsequent risk of breast cancer in half. If lowered estrogen levels following removal of the ovaries were the reason for the drop in breast cancer risk, as many oncologists believed, giving these women supplemental estrogen to alleviate symptoms of menopause would be illogical; indeed, it would be dangerously risky. But it isn't. The investigators compared BRCA-positive women who had been taking HRT or ERT for a few years following removal of their ovaries with those who had never taken hormones and found no increased risk of breast cancer.[22] Neither did Andrea Eisen, a medical oncologist at the Sunnybrook Regional Cancer Center in Toronto, who studied 472 BRCA1-positive postmenopausal women, half of whom were taking hormones and half of whom were not. She concluded that "among postmenopausal women with a BRCA1 mutation, estrogen use, which averaged around 4 years, was not associated with an increased risk of breast cancer; *indeed, in this population, it was associated with a significant decreased risk*"[23] [emphasis ours]. This result was replicated in 2016 in a multicenter report by Joanne

Kotsopoulos, a research scientist who studies breast and ovarian cancer at the School of Public Health at the University of Toronto; again, women with a BRCA1 mutation who had been on HRT for an average of 4.3 years had no increased risk of breast cancer.[24]

At this point, you might be saying to yourself, "Why would anyone ever think that estrogen increases the risk of breast cancer?" We thought you'd never ask.

Those who make the case for the dangers of hormones cite two studies in particular to bolster their argument. One was published in 1989 in the *NEJM* by a team of eminent researchers, led by Leif Bergkvist and Hans-Olov Adami of the department of surgery at University Hospital, Uppsala, Sweden. It reported a frightening result: a 440 percent increased risk of breast cancer among women who had been on HRT.[25] This article continues to be cited as evidence for the dangers of HRT.

So let's look at that study. The researchers analyzed prescription forms from the entire female population around Uppsala who were on ERT or HRT—more than twenty-three thousand women. Instead of going through the records of all of those women, which would have been a time-consuming challenge, they selected a subgroup of that large sample, one in every thirty or so, and ended up with 638 women who filled out their two sequential questionnaires. They found no increased risk of breast cancer among women taking estrogen alone. Among an unspecified, smaller number of the 638 patients who were taking estrogen and progestin, the authors had calculated that 2.2 breast cancers would be expected. Instead, breast cancer developed in 10 women—a 440 percent increase in risk. With numbers that small, the increase could have been a statistical fluke, and in fact the researchers admitted that their result was not statistically significant. We repeat: not statistically significant! But because this was the lead article in the *New England Journal of Medicine,* many physicians went to town over the 440 percent, trumpeting that "increased risk" as if it were meaningful. In a study published not long after their first one, the same authors actually reported a better prognosis among breast cancer patients who were on estrogen at the time of diagnosis than among those who were not.[26]

In an editorial accompanying that first paper in the *NEJM,* Elizabeth Barrett-Connor, a biomedical scientist and professor in the departments of family medicine and public health at the University of California, San Diego, wrote: "For the average North American woman, who will be postmenopausal for one third of her life, the benefits of estrogen seem strongly established. In my opinion, the data are not conclusive enough to warrant any immediate change in the way we approach hormone replacement."[27] The *Harvard Medical School Health Letter* also reviewed the Swedish study and concluded that the difference between 2.2 and 10 patients was too small to provide a statistically stable result, let alone one that warranted overturning most of the earlier research that "has given us no reason to expect a strong association between estrogen replacement and breast cancer."[28]

The second big study cited by those who think HRT is unsafe was published in 1997 in the *Lancet.* This was the Collaborative Reanalysis, a survey of fifty-one epidemiological studies from twenty-one countries involving 52,705 women with breast cancer and 108,411 women without breast cancer. Because of the study's enormous size and the reputation of its more than twenty collaborators (many of whom could be included in a Who's Who of cancer research), it is still frequently cited as one of *the* definitive investigations of hormones and breast cancer. The researchers—led by epidemiologists Richard Doll, Richard Peto, and Valerie Beral of the project's analysis and writing committee—reported no increase in breast cancer among women who had taken HRT in the past, no matter how long they had taken it. Did the researchers then say, "Good news!" and move on? No; they reanalyzed their voluminous data to see if they could find, anywhere, a subgroup of women who showed an increased risk of breast cancer associated with HRT. They found it by extracting the women who were still on HRT at the time they were interviewed and who had been on it for five or more years.[29] How small an increase did they find? Even in this artificially constructed sample, the increased number of breast cancers in one hundred women taking estrogen for ten or more years was 0.6, less than one additional case.[30]

And that's where matters stood until 2002.

Enter the Women's Health Initiative

In July 2002, the National Institutes of Health issued a press release that immediately got the attention of every medical journalist around the world: "The National Heart, Lung, and Blood Institute of the NIH has stopped early the Women's Health Initiative, a major clinical trial of the risks and benefits of combined estrogen and progestin in healthy menopausal women due to an increased risk of invasive breast cancer." This press release was followed by one from the *Journal of the American Medical Association* in advance of its publishing the paper: "Hormone Therapy Study Stopped Due to Increased Breast Cancer Risk." *JAMA* added that the study was stopped not only because of increased breast cancer risk, but also because of increased risks of "coronary heart disease, stroke, and pulmonary embolisms."

These press releases generated an avalanche of excited headlines: "HRT Linked to Breast Cancer," announced the BBC. "Hormone Replacement Study a Shock to the Medical System," said the *New York Times*, which quoted Wulf Utian, an obstetrician-gynecologist who was also executive director of the North American Menopause Society: "This is the biggest bombshell that ever hit in my 30-something years in the menopause area."

It certainly was. The WHI was the largest prospective study in which women were randomized to take either hormones or a placebo and then followed over time.[31] This method is considered the gold standard of scientific research, because if you simply compare women who choose to take estrogen with those who choose not to—as many earlier studies did—you can't say whether estrogen makes women healthier or if healthier women take estrogen.* The WHI cost nearly one billion dollars; its investigators were leading physicians, statisticians, and epidemiologists across the country; and the findings were published in medicine's most prestigious journals. No wonder the announcement caused a panic among the millions of women taking hormones, and no wonder the prescription rate for HRT fell by up to 70 percent within a short time.[32] Confusion trailed panic; *Newsweek* summed it up in a long article headlined "What's a

---

* Nevertheless, reviews of the medical literature comparing results from observational studies with those from randomized controlled trials have found that both methods often produce similar outcomes. We will discuss this important concern further in chapters 3 and 8.

Woman to Do?" Should women who have menopausal symptoms deny themselves the benefits of HRT, in the short term or over many years, because they fear breast cancer, heart disease, or stroke? Are their concerns warranted by the WHI's claims?

Let's start with the claim about breast cancer. The WHI investigators reported that women who were randomly assigned to take estrogen on its own had had no increased risk of breast cancer. Those who still had a uterus and were assigned to take the combination of estrogen and progestin had a small increased risk of breast cancer (1.26) when compared with women who were randomly assigned to a placebo. That number, 1.26, would mean a 26 percent increase in risk. What few noticed was this sentence: "The 26 percent increase in breast cancer incidence among the HRT group compared with the placebo group almost reached nominal statistical significance." *Almost* means it did *not* reach statistical significance, and that means it could have been a spurious association. (Scientists have arbitrarily agreed that the results of a study are not considered statistically significant unless the probability that its results are due to chance alone is less than one in twenty.) Of course, any increase might be of legitimate concern and warrant further investigation. Yet many reporters and physicians treated that 26 percent increase in risk as being not only statistically significant but also medically significant.

Garnet Anderson, co–principal investigator and biostatistician for the WHI Clinical Coordinating Center, claimed the study had demonstrated that "breast cancer rates were markedly increased among women assigned to the estrogen plus progestin group."[33] Markedly? Even if this finding had been statistically significant, which it was not, it would have meant that HRT increased the risk of breast cancer from five women in one hundred to six in one hundred. (And recall that women diagnosed with breast cancer while taking HRT have a better prognosis than women diagnosed in the absence of HRT.) In the WHI's press release, Anderson justified her statistical decisions this way: "Because breast cancer is so serious an event, we set the bar lower to monitor for it. We pre-specified that the change in cancer rates did not have to be that large to warrant stopping the trial. And the trial was stopped at the first clear indication of increased risk."

In other words: *We set the bar low enough to monitor for nonsignificant results if we could squeak out any.*

The WHI researchers continued to follow the patients from the original study, updating their data set as those patients stayed healthy or developed illnesses. A year later, in 2003, they reported that the small difference in breast cancer incidence between patients randomized to HRT and those randomized to placebo had narrowed, but, curiously, it now barely achieved statistical significance. Still, they asserted that their 2002 report "confirmed that combined estrogen plus progestin use increases the risk of invasive breast cancer."[34]

In 2006, in another update of this same cohort of women, the WHI reported that they found no increased risk of breast cancer among those same women randomized to combined estrogen-progestin treatment.[35] The alleged increased risk—the one worth stopping the study for—had completely vanished. This news did not make headlines. As the science writer Tara Parker-Pope noted in her 2007 book *The Hormone Decision,* the WHI "seemed to have a different standard for bad hormone news than it did for good hormone news."[36]

The WHI continued their campaign of fear for the next dozen

years. In 2008 they reported that among the women who had received HRT, even years after they stopped taking it, the death rate from all causes was "somewhat higher than among those assigned to placebo"—even though this difference in mortality, once again, did not reach statistical significance. This nonsignificant increase in mortality, they added, "was accounted for by deaths attributed to various cancers unrelated to the pre-specified trial outcomes…most prominently lung cancer."[37] What? No increased mortality from breast cancer, and suddenly we are talking about lung cancer? (Not to worry; they subsequently dropped that concern.)

In 2010 the WHI authors published yet another article, this one claiming that women who had been on HRT suffered more deaths from breast cancer (2.6 versus 1.3 deaths per 10,000 women per year) than those who had been on a placebo—again, a difference that was not statistically significant.[38]

The WHI was heralded as being truly representative of women during and after menopause, and the WHI investigators repeatedly stated that all of the women they recruited were healthy at the outset of the study, but neither assertion was true. Fully 35 percent of the women were considerably overweight, and another 34 percent were obese; nearly 36 percent were being treated for high blood pressure; nearly half were either current or past cigarette smokers.[39] Moreover, the median age of participants was sixty-three, long past the onset of menopause. Therefore, there is no credible reason for generalizing from the results of this study to the entire population of postmenopausal women—even though that was precisely what this randomized controlled study was supposed to do.

In recent years, medical researchers have become more vocal in their critical reassessment of the WHI's methods, findings, and conclusions. As one prominent example, in 2014, Samuel Shapiro, then in the department of public health and family medicine at the University of Cape Town Medical School, and his colleagues conducted an in-depth statistical analysis and concluded that "the over-interpretation and misrepresentation of the findings in the WHI study has resulted in major damage to the health and well-being of menopausal women. The WHI was not 'a victory for women and their health,' and the claim that 'the findings do not support the use of this therapy for chronic disease prevention' is not defensible. Nor can the pejorative editorial statement that 'the WHI overturned medical dogma regarding menopausal hormone therapy' be defended."[40]

But the most damning indictment of the WHI was yet to come—from one of its principal investigators. In March 2017, Robert Langer, associate dean for clinical and translational research at the University of Nevada, published an insider's view. He wrote: "Highly unusual circumstances prevailed when the WHI trial was stopped prematurely in July 2002. The investigators most capable of correcting the critical misinterpretations of the data were actively excluded from the writing and dissemination activities." Actively excluded! The paper of initial results, he said, was written by a small group in the WHI program office who submitted it to the medical journal without informing the principal investigators. He described what happened at the meeting of the principal investigators and the NIH program staff:

The investigator group was stunned by the announcement that the Data Safety and Monitoring Committee had recommended stopping the estrogen-progestin trial and that the director had accepted their recommendation. Minutes later the group was shocked by the distribution of a typeset copy of the primary results paper soon to be published in *JAMA*. *This was the first time that the vast majority of principal investigators had seen the paper* [emphasis ours]. The meeting was paused so that we could read it. Some of us were aghast. Concerns were raised about the propriety of producing a paper on behalf of the entire study group in this manner. More importantly, concerns were raised about the tone, the analyses conducted and reported, and the interpretation of the results in the paper.[41]

The protesting investigators were allowed to do some quick editing of the article before lunch, addressing its "tone and interpretation," and the changes were sent by courier to *JAMA*. They were too late. The courier returned to tell them that the issue had already been printed and was in the warehouses ready to be mailed out.

In short, the procedure violated key scientific conventions: statistical accuracy, co-author review, and publication in a professional journal *before* the hoopla of press releases and other publicity. Jacques Rossouw, a cardiologist who was a principal investigator of the WHI, told Parker-Pope that the WHI "was intentionally going for 'high impact' when it called the press conference," because they didn't want their news to "get lost in the shuffle of daily news events," especially when their goal "was to shake up the medical establishment and change the thinking about hormones."[42]

And that is the giveaway. Far from setting out to do an unbiased study to investigate the possible benefits and risks of hormones for women during and after menopause, far from their disingenuous claims that they fully expected to learn that hormones were safe, some of the principal investigators had an agenda from the outset: to "change the thinking about hormones" and show that they were harmful. After the WHI had begun but six years before any findings were published, Rossouw had published a paper in which he lamented the widespread use of estrogen.[43] "The bandwagon [in support of estrogen replacement therapy] is clearly rolling," he wrote, "as anyone who reads newspapers or magazines, watches television, or talks to colleagues can attest. The bandwagon appears to be picking up in speed and volume. The putative benefits of HRT are being trumpeted to postmenopausal women, with only transient muting for reports of possible adverse effects." It is time, Rossouw argued, to put "the brakes on that bandwagon." The WHI certainly did.

The WHI and *JAMA* might have been justified in bypassing scientific conventions if the findings were truly of enormous medical import, but they were not. Instead, the investigators collaborated in generating international panic based on data and conclusions that were open to serious question. Why did they do this? Along with Rossouw, they clearly felt that the pro-HRT bandwagon was perilously out of control. In 2002, a few months after the WHI's first stop-the-presses report was published, one of its principal investigators spoke about the study at the continuing medical education program that Av was running at his hospital. A number of physicians in the audience were not impressed by the borderline or not statistically significant evidence being presented, and the following exchange during the question-and-answer period was recorded:

Physician: About your claim of the increased risk of breast cancer for women on HRT, I'm not an oncologist so this might be a stupid question. I was under the impression that if the confidence interval [a measure of a finding's strength] included the number one, that it was not particularly meaningful.

WHI Investigator: Yeah, yeah, you know, that's right. And you know what happens? What happens is, if it's an important question and if it's a big study…and you can't do it again because it costs too much money, then they'll say that's the best data there is and then [inaudible] the statistical police have to leave the room. So that's the answer.

Translation: We won't ever be able to do this study again. We know, we just know in our heart of hearts, that HRT is harmful and causes breast cancer. And even if not cancer so much, then other diseases for sure. Therefore, if we get ambiguous answers or nonsignificant ones, we ask the statistical police to leave the room.

ENTER THE MILLION WOMEN STUDY: RUMMAGING FOR RISKS

A year after the WHI exploded on the medical landscape, another enormous project generated headlines that added to women's worries. The Million Women Study, a British study published in the *Lancet,* reported an increased risk of breast cancer in women taking ERT or HRT.[44] However, this increased risk occurred only in women currently taking hormones, with no increased risk in past users of either estrogen or estrogen-progestin, regardless of how long they had been on either. Readers who are thinking *Huh?* right about now are not alone. If estrogen is a major risk factor in breast cancer, why would *having taken it for years* not be a problem but *taking it at the time of the study* be a risk?

The WHI and the Million Women Study, like many other efforts to identify the causes of disease, committed two statistical errors. One has to do with how risks are reported; the other has to do with a statistical manipulation called *data mining*. Stay with us here, because this information could improve your life—maybe even save it.

Consider, first, the difference between absolute risk and relative risk. The media, following the example of many researchers themselves, tend to report relative risks, which are expressed in percentages that can seem more important than they are. For example, if you learn that the relative risk of breast cancer is increased by 300 percent in women who eat a bagel every morning, that sounds serious, but it is not informative. You would need to know the baseline absolute number of new breast cancer patients in women who avoid bagels. If the number of new cases in bagel-avoiders was 1 in 10,000 women and the number of new cases in bagel-eaters was 3 in 10,000 women, that *is* a 300 percent increase, but it is very likely a random result—enjoy your bagel! If the risk jumped from 100 new cases in 10,000 bagel-avoiders to 300 new cases in 10,000 bagel-eaters, also a 300 percent increase, you might reasonably be concerned and cut down on your bagel consumption.

In epidemiological studies, which generally include tens of thousands of people, it is easy to find a small relationship that may be considered significant by statistical convention but that, in practical terms, means little or nothing because of the low absolute numbers.[45] This is why scientists who are working to promote statistical literacy, especially by helping the public and physicians understand actual versus inflated risks of diseases and treatments, emphasize that knowing the baseline of absolute numbers when comparing two groups is essential.[46] Throughout this book, we too will be reporting results that showed such-and-such a reduction (or increase) in risk, but we have taken pains wherever possible to ensure that these numbers reflect meaningful findings in absolute terms, not trivial ones. Thus, we will not cite a study if it reported a 33 percent reduction in risk if that reduction was from 3 to 2. We say "wherever possible" because, regrettably, sometimes it isn't possible to know the absolute numbers in a published study because of how the numbers are presented.

Many of the studies of HRT and risk of disease, especially breast cancer, have produced statistically modest or borderline results that have been made to look more impressive than they really are because researchers report only relative risks. In 2003, the WHI claimed that HRT increased women's risk of breast cancer by 24 percent; in 2002, it was 26 percent. Does that percentage really merit international headlines? The table following lists the reported decreases and increases in relative risks associated not only with ERT and HRT but also many other things, such as stress causing a decreased risk or chewing betel quid causing an increased risk. You can see at a glance how weak and probably meaningless these associations are. To put them in perspective, the last entry is a truly important and meaningful link: the one between tobacco smoking and lung cancer.

Risk Factors Reported to Be Associated with Breast Cancer [47]

Risk Factor	Relative Risk*
Dietary fiber intake	0.31
Significant weight gain from age 21 to present	0.52
Garlic and onions 7 to 10 times a week	0.52
High level of stress	0.60
Grapefruit	0.60
Fish oil	0.68
Large body build at menarche	0.69
Conjugated equine estrogen (Premarin)	0.77
Aspirin	0.80
Coffee consumption more than 5 cups a day	0.80
Above average weight at the age of 12	0.85
Low income	0.85
Fish intake	1.14
Birth length greater than 20 inches	1.17
Use of antihypertensive medication for more than 5 years	1.18
Multivitamin use	1.19
Exposure to light at night	1.22
Premarin/progestin (WHI, 2003)	1.24
Premarin/progestin (WHI, 2002)	1.26
Alcohol	1.26
French fries (1 additional serving per week during preschool years)	1.27
Physical abuse in adulthood	1.28
Grapefruit (again)	1.30
Digoxin (current users)	1.39
Night-shift work	1.51

More than 15 kg weight gain during pregnancy	1.61
Flight attendant (Finnish)	1.87
Father at least 40 years old at patient's birth (premenopausal breast cancer)	1.90
Exposed to Dutch famine, 1944–1945, only between ages 2 and 9 at the time	2.01
Placental weight	2.05
Antibiotic use for more than 1,001 days	2.07
Increased carbohydrate intake	2.22
Calcium channel blocker for more than 10 years	2.40
Left-handedness (premenopausal)	2.41
Flight attendant (Icelandic)	4.10
Betel-quid chewing	4.78
Electric-blanket use	4.90

And here's a statistical association that actually means something:

Tobacco smoking and lung cancer	26.07

* A relative risk of 1 means there is no effect on risk. A relative risk of less than 1 means an associated decreased risk, and a relative risk of greater than 1 means an increased risk.

Another way of misrepresenting findings comes from the practice, severely frowned upon in research, of retrospective substratification, commonly known as data mining. Data mining occurs when researchers, having failed to find a statistically significant association that they had hypothesized would exist between a possible risk factor and a disease, go back into their data and rummage around, looking for other factors that might show a statistical link. This effort might yield interesting questions or hypotheses for future research, but the problem is that in a data set of many thousands of people, some relationships that are unearthed retrospectively will turn out to be statistically significant but meaningless. In *Against the Gods: The Remarkable Story of Risk,* the economist Peter Bernstein put it this way: "If you torture the data long enough, the numbers will prove anything you want."[48]

A now-famous example of the spurious results that can emerge from data mining can be found in an article that was submitted to the *Lancet* in 1988. It reported that men hospitalized for acute heart attacks who had been taking a daily aspirin had a better survival rate than similar men who had not been on aspirin. This was obviously an important finding, and the editors agreed to accept this article with one condition: the authors would have to retrospectively substratify the 17,187 men in their study according to a variety of factors, including the men's ages, weights, and races.

Now, it would certainly be good to know if the benefit of taking aspirin (or any other drug) is affected by being old, overweight, Italian, a yoga practitioner, an owner of a 1968 red Camaro, or other demographic factors. But the authors correctly refused to do this reanalysis, explaining that it would be bad science and that the benefit or risk for these subcategories would best be assessed by a new prospective study.[49] The editors insisted—no substratification, no publication.

And so the authors eventually turned in a revised article with the additional findings, plus one more: a slight adverse effect of aspirin on mortality in patients born under the astrological signs of Gemini and Libra in contrast to a strikingly beneficial effect of aspirin for patients born under all other astrological signs. The editors agreed to publish the article if the astrological results were omitted. "You wanted retrospective substratification, we gave you retrospective substratification," the authors said (in effect), and they demanded that the journal stick to the deal. And so this landmark article was published, explaining aspirin's effect on "myocardial infarct mortality" among men born under the signs of Gemini and Libra, the latter subgroup analysis clearly not being taken seriously in the article.[50] One scientist titled his commentary on this study "Subgroup analyses in clinical trials: Fun to look at—but don't believe them!" He wrote: "Of course most physicians (but not all!) laughed when they were presented with these results. However, when presented with other less ridiculous subgroup analyses they are likely to believe the results, and forget the example from astrology, particularly if the result can be justified by some pet theory."[51]

Here's how researchers who have the best of intentions—and a pet theory—can get caught up in data mining. We showed how this happened in the Million Women Study, but even the highly respected Nurses' Health Study, referred to earlier, can make this mistake. The Nurses' Health Study followed 121,700 female registered nurses for decades and reported no increase in breast cancer among the women who had used HRT at any point, even if they'd been on it for more than ten years. Instead of being satisfied, the investigators substratified their patients into two groups: (1) women who had been taking hormones for at least five years and were still doing so, and (2) women who had taken hormones in the past and had stopped. This time they found an increased risk of breast cancer, but only among women who were currently on ERT or HRT and had been taking it for at least five years.[52]

Think for a moment how unlikely this is. If, as many of those who oppose the use of HRT believe, lifetime exposure to estrogen is associated with an increasing risk of breast cancer—the more estrogen, the higher the risk — how can you get an increased risk among a group of women who have taken hormones for five years but not among those who took it for more than ten years? Can you think of any other documented cause of cancer (for example, tobacco or asbestos) that carries more risk if you are currently exposed to it and have been for a relatively brief time and less risk if you are not currently exposed to it but you were for many years in the past? Neither can we. That is what data mining gives you.

Consider this study from the National Cancer Institute, published in *JAMA* in 2000, reporting on a follow-up of 2,082 women with breast cancer that also found no increase in risk associated with ERT. The increased risk associated with HRT was restricted to those who used hormones during the four years prior to diagnosis and who weighed ninety pounds or less. That's what data mining gives you.[53]

Or how about the finding in the table on page 38 that using an electric blanket increases the risk of breast cancer? That finding was significant only for African American women, only if they used electric blankets for more than ten years — and only when those who used blankets for more than six months per year were excluded! That's what data mining gives you.

Some investigators who believe that the relative risks of HRT are serious enough to warrant concern acknowledge that the absolute risks from this treatment are small — increasing a woman's risk by no more than 2 percent.[54] Moreover, even if HRT increases the risk of breast cancer by this modest fraction, other research suggests that women on HRT live longer than those not taking it and have a lower death rate from breast cancer.[55] How can the very hormones that allegedly increase the risk of breast cancer also be responsible for better survival from that cancer?

Does Estrogen Cause Breast Cancer? How Would We Know?

In medicine, as in law, causation is often difficult to prove beyond a reasonable doubt. A bullet fired through the brain or the heart of an otherwise healthy human being who dies shortly thereafter generally provides both a necessary and sufficient explanation for the cause of death. But many causes of disease and death are not as straightforward; they are inferred and then must be tested and confirmed—or rejected.

Consider the effort to find the cause of tuberculosis. Because tuberculosis was often concentrated in large metropolitan areas, physicians originally believed it was caused by the stress of living in crowded, noisy spaces. Accordingly, throughout the United States and Europe, tuberculosis sanitariums were set up to remove affected individuals from their allegedly stressful environments. In these peaceful sanitariums, patients were even placed in dark rooms with window shades lowered to further decrease stress. Thomas Mann's *The Magic Mountain* describes just such an environment.

In 1872 Robert Koch demonstrated unequivocally that the cause of tuberculosis was the tubercle bacillus, and only then were the sanitariums gradually closed and antibiotics developed to treat this scourge. To prove the role of the tubercle bacillus, Koch set up four postulates, and these have served as a template for the study of the causes of other human diseases.[56] Koch's postulates—the steps needed to demonstrate that microorganism A is indeed the cause of disease B—were as follows:

- The microorganism must be found in all organisms suffering from the disease.
- The microorganism must be isolated from a diseased organism and grown in pure culture.
- The cultured microorganism should cause the disease when introduced into a healthy organism.
- The microorganism must be re-isolated from the inoculated diseased host and shown to be the same as the original causative agent.

This causal *chain of evidence* is now an established format for determining causation in medicine. A famous example is the discovery of the bacterium *H. pylori* as the cause of gastritis and peptic ulcers during an era when ulcers were thought to be caused by stress (a popular villain for many diseases), suppressed anger, or spicy food. In the early 1980s Australian pathologist Robin Warren and Australian physician Barry Marshall finally succeeded in culturing the bacteria from the stomach (by accident, actually; they had unintentionally left their petri dishes incubating for five days over a holiday weekend). Their paper arguing that *H. pylori* was the culprit, forget anger and Thai food, initially met with resistance and skepticism, but within a few years other researchers verified the association of the bacteria with gastritis and ulcers. Then, to demonstrate that *H. pylori* was the cause and that the association was not merely coincidental, Marshall offered up his body to science. He drank a beaker of *H. pylori* culture and within a few days became ill with nausea and vomiting. Subsequent tests confirmed signs of gastritis and the presence of *H. pylori*. Marshall and Warren went on to demonstrate that antibiotics are effective in the treatment of many cases of gastritis and ulcers. Their work was recognized with a Nobel Prize.

The causal chain is only as strong as its weakest link, and disproving a single item of evidence can overthrow the entire hypothesis. That is why Koch's postulates function best in the field of microbiology. You can't apply them in the field of epidemiology, the arena, as science writer Gary Taubes explained, where most controversies about causation in health and disease take place.[57] Epidemiologists try to identify patterns and correlations across studies of different and often enormous populations, and their conclusions rest on whatever statistical associations emerge. But as statisticians and college teachers forever try to impress on students and laypeople, *correlation does not imply causation.* Two things may be statistically correlated but in reality have nothing to do with each other. The number of storks nesting in certain European villages is reportedly correlated with the number of babies born in those villages, but (as far as we know) storks don't bring babies, and babies don't attract storks. It's just that human births are more frequent at certain times of year, and those peaks happen to coincide with the storks' nesting periods.

Storks and babies are an example of an illusory correlation, an apparent association between two things that is merely coincidental. Illusory correlations can create dangerous beliefs and cause great social harm. Claims of an association between autism and vaccination for childhood diseases alarmed many parents, but study after study has failed to find any connection whatsoever. In one major study of all children born in Denmark between 1991 and 1998 (over half a million children), the incidence of autism in vaccinated children was a bit lower than in unvaccinated children. The apparent link between vaccination and autism is almost certainly a coincidence, an illusory correlation, arising from the fact that symptoms of childhood autism are often first recognized at about the same time that children get a series of vaccines.[58]

Because of the problem of illusory correlations—as well as the statistical likelihood that in a sample of many thousands of people, some correlations will occur just by chance—epidemiological evidence in determining the cause of a disease cannot be as scientifically rigorous as Koch's postulates. Epidemiological studies form a *mosaic* of scattered findings rather than a linked chain. Unlike with a chain, which can be broken by one weak link, cutting out one piece of a mosaic may weaken the overall picture but it will not destroy it. Contradictory findings simply alter the balance of probability that a hypothesis is correct.[59]

By understanding the mosaic created by epidemiological studies, we can see why so many medical hypotheses persist long after they have been disconfirmed and why so many studies in health and medicine keep contradicting one another—to the exasperation of the public. Well, *should* I get B_{12} injections? Well, *is* coffee harmful? Once you told me that margarine was healthier than butter and now you tell me that butter is better. Well, which is it?*

It is true that on rare occasions, correlational evidence may be strong enough to support causation. In 1775, a British surgeon with the wonderful name of Percivall Pott noticed a marked rise in cases of scrotal cancer in his clinic, almost invariably in young chimney sweeps. When two rare events strongly intersect, the

---

* Only if you are seriously deficient in vitamin B_{12}. Coffee is fine. Butter is better.

association between them implies causality. And, indeed, chimney sweeping and scrotal cancer were both uncommon enough that the overlap between the two stood out starkly, and Pott could safely infer that chimney sweeping increased the risk of scrotal cancer. Eventually, that inference was scientifically confirmed, and Pott became the first scientist to demonstrate that a cancer may be caused by an environmental carcinogen. Such a convincing association between rare events, however, is the exception.

How, then, should we approach the mosaic of findings that occur with more complicated diseases, such as breast cancer?

The Physician as Detective

Austin Bradford Hill, the British biostatistician who pioneered the randomized clinical trial in the 1940s, offered an answer. He suggested that a case for causation in epidemiology, unlike in microbiology, should be structured in the same way a detective proves a case: the preponderance of pieces of evidence, rather than a single definitive experiment, establishes cause.[60] In 1965, he proposed nine "viewpoints" (which came to be referred to as the Bradford Hill criteria) that he suggested could help scientists determine whether there is a causal relationship between the proposed agent and the specific disease. Let's look at the eight most relevant to our story.*

---

* We are omitting his ninth one, judging by analogy, because it was the vaguest and most disputed. As noted in a recent textbook, "Whatever insight might be derived from analogy is handicapped by the inventive imagination of scientists who can find analogies everywhere" (K. J. Rothman, S. Greenland, and T. L. Lash, *Modern Epidemiology* [Philadelphia: Wolters Kluwer, 2012], 30).

Strength: The evidence must be strong; that is, statistically significant and not trivially so.

Consistency: The evidence must be consistent across different studies and populations.

Specificity: When a risk factor or cause produces a specific result, it adds support for the hypothesis. In epidemiology, it is often difficult to achieve such specificity, because the spread and incidence of a disease is frequently a result of many factors, but the absence of specificity supports the inference that A is not the cause of B.

Temporal relationship: Exposure to the risk factor always precedes the outcome.

Dose-response relationship: Hill called this a biological gradient, meaning that an increased dose of or exposure to the risk factor should lead to increased incidence of the disease, and, conversely, the incidence of the disease should decline when exposure to the factor is reduced or eliminated.

Plausibility: The evidence and the theory behind it must be plausible, agreeing with the currently accepted understanding of the disease-causing processes. A chance correlation, as between shoe size and flute-playing ability, is implausible.

Coherence: The association between factor A and disease B should be compatible with existing knowledge. Of course, a new theory and supporting data can overturn an orthodox assumption and cause a paradigm shift. But if a hypothesis or belief—say, that the world was created six thousand years ago or that giraffes can levitate—requires a major sacrifice of everything known about archaeology, physics, biology, and anthropology, that theory is likely to be invalid.

Experiment: The disease can be prevented or ameliorated by a particular experimental intervention.

Finally, we want to add a ninth criterion: consideration of *alternative explanations,* which is a fundamental ingredient of the scientific method. Before concluding that A causes B or that A increases the risk of B, scientists must consider other possible explanations of B and rule them out.

The relationship between cigarette smoking and lung cancer is a good example of a convincing mosaic of evidence. The causal relationship meets all of Hill's criteria:

Strength: The data show a 1,000 to 3,000 percent increase in the risk of lung cancer in smokers compared to nonsmokers.

Consistency: The strong association between cigarette smoking and lung cancer has been confirmed in most, if not all, studies.

Specificity: Eighty-five percent of all lung cancer patients are or were smokers. Some lung cancer patients, although nonsmokers, were exposed to secondhand smoke, a possible risk factor for the disease.

Temporal relationship: The practice of smoking precedes development of the disease (apart from the minority of cases in which the nonsmoking patient had a genetic predisposition or exposure to other carcinogens).

Dose-response relationship: The more cigarettes that people smoke and the more years they smoke, the greater their risk of lung cancer.

Plausibility: Cigarette smoke has been shown to cause premalignant changes in the lungs of laboratory animals. Similar changes have been seen in the lungs of smokers, including those who later developed lung cancer.

Coherence: The association between smoking and lung cancer conforms to existing physiological research and theory.

Experiment: As rates of smoking and exposure to secondhand smoke have declined, so have rates of lung cancer. Conversely, as rates of smoking rose among women, so did rates of lung cancer.

Alternative explanations: Other risk factors in lung cancer have been ruled out or understood to apply in only a minority of cases.

Now let's consider hormones—specifically estrogen—and breast cancer. Using Hill's framework, is the link between estrogen and breast cancer supported?

Strength: The link is unsupported. Most of the correlations published by the WHI and other investigators were neither strong nor statistically significant by conventional standards.

Consistency: The link is unsupported. Most published reports find no consistently increased risk of breast cancer associated with ERT. On the contrary, the results could not be more inconsistent: Between 1975 and 2000, forty-five published studies examined the relationship between breast cancer and ERT. Of these, 82 percent found no increased risk; 13 percent found a very small increased risk; and 5 percent found a decreased risk. In that same twenty-five-year period, of twenty published studies of HRT, 80 percent found no increased risk, 10 percent found an increased risk, and 10 percent found a decreased risk.[61]

Specificity: The link is unsupported. The overwhelming majority of breast cancer patients have never taken estrogen, and the vast majority of women who have taken hormones have never developed breast cancer.

Temporal relationship: The link is unsupported. Taking estrogen does not always, or even frequently, precede the onset of the disease. The risk of breast cancer increases with age—even after menopause, when estrogen declines, and even among women who never took estrogen.[62]

Dose-response relationship: The link is unsupported. Study after study finds no consistent increased risk of breast cancer in women who have taken ERT or HRT for five years, ten years, or fifteen years. If cumulative exposure to estrogen is a risk factor in breast cancer, why did the Nurses' Health Study and the Million Women Study find that risk only among current users rather than past users? Some investigators assert that early menarche and late menopause, which would provide a woman with more exposure to estrogen in her lifetime, are associated with an increased risk of breast cancer. But they are not. Four separate studies have examined the breast cancer risks to women who started their periods between the ages of twelve and seventeen as compared to the risks for women whose periods started at age eleven or younger. In two of these studies, no differences in risk were found. In the other two, a significant reduction in risk was found only among women who started their periods at age seventeen and older; but they, like those whose menarche began before age eleven, represent a very small outlying percentage of the population. None of the comparisons for any of the other ages resulted in differences that were significant in any of the four studies.[63]

Plausibility: The link is unsupported. Surely, the most disconfirming evidence for the claim that estrogen causes breast cancer is this: the administration of estrogen has been shown to have beneficial effects even in women with advanced breast cancer. For example, in 1944 Sir Alexander Haddow, director of the Institute for Cancer Research at the University of London, reported that 25 percent of his patients with advanced breast cancer improved when given high-dose estrogen,[64] and other researchers subsequently have gotten the same or better results. Oncologist Bruno Massidda and his team at the University of Cagliari, Italy, reported remission in 50 percent of advanced breast cancer patients treated with estrogens,[65] and so did Reshma Mahtani and colleagues at the Boca Raton Comprehensive Cancer Center.[66] Gabriel N. Hortobagyi and colleagues at the MD Anderson Cancer Center reported that the most effective therapy for metastatic carcinoma of the breast was combined estrogen-progestin.[67] James Ingle and colleagues at the Mayo Clinic demonstrated better survival among breast cancer patients treated with diethylstilbestrol (DES), a form of estrogen, compared to tamoxifen,[68] as did Per Eystein Lønning and colleagues at Haukeland University Hospital in Norway.[69] And the pioneer cancer researcher V. Craig Jordan and his research team demonstrated that both high and low doses of estrogen can shrink cancerous breast tumors.[70]

Coherence: The link is unsupported. Using the mosaic method of knowledge, the more pieces we add, the clearer the overall image should become. That is what happened in confirming the relationship between smoking and lung cancer, and it is precisely what has *not* happened in the persistent efforts to confirm a relationship between estrogen and breast cancer.

Experiment: The link is unsupported. In 1999, breast cancer rates began to decline. The WHI investigators claimed credit, maintaining that thanks to their 2002 warning that HRT was a cause of breast cancer, the number of women taking hormones plummeted—and thus did not develop breast cancer. However, their claim had several fundamental flaws. First, the decline began three years before the WHI published anything. Second, in Sweden and Norway, women stopped taking HRT at about the same rate that American women did but had no additional drop in rates of breast cancer.[71] And third, because breast cancer usually takes years to become clinically detectable, how could a drop in the rate of breast cancer be related to stopping HRT one year prior? The WHI authors responded by saying that's because when women went off estrogen, they removed a stimulus to the growth of *already present but not yet detectable (subclinical)* breast cancer.[72] If that were so, however, the decreased incidence should have been confined to small, early, non-invasive breast cancers; it was not. It occurred almost entirely with invasive breast cancers.[73]

Alternative explanations: Not ruled out. When researchers fail to confirm their hypothesized link between risk factor A and disease B, they are then supposed to consider other explanations and explore other risk factors. But over and over in the studies of estrogen and breast cancer, we see researchers unable to accept their own evidence of small, weak, contradictory, or nonexistent links. Instead of considering alternative explanations, they have often resorted to data mining or retrospective substratification to try to find *something* somewhere in the data that supports their belief that a significant association must be in there.

Bradford Hill ended his 1965 paper by saying, "All scientific work is incomplete—whether it be observational or experimental. All scientific work is liable to be upset or modified by advancing knowledge. That does not confer upon us a freedom to ignore the knowledge we already have, or to postpone the action that it appears to demand at a given time."

THE TAKE-HOME

In sum, the hypothesis that estrogen is a real risk factor in breast cancer fails to meet Austin Bradford Hill's criteria. Why, then, has the belief that estrogen causes breast cancer persisted?

The tobacco industry fought the data showing a link between tobacco and lung cancer with a powerful weapon: doubt. An unpublished tobacco industry report drawn up in 1969 stated their strategy explicitly: "Doubt is our product, since it is the best means of competing with the body of fact."[74] But anti-smoking advocates had their own weapon, something just as visceral: fear—and fear of the most terrifying illness, cancer. Today, the reports linking HRT to breast cancer rely on fear rather than doubt to fortify their arguments, perhaps because doubt does not generate as much attention or emotion. But the fear of HRT is misplaced. After all, the percentage of lung cancer patients who were smokers is approximately 85 percent, and the current cure rate for lung cancer is approximately 15 percent. By contrast, the percentage of breast cancer patients who have ever used HRT is 11 to 24 percent, and the 2018 cure rate for newly diagnosed breast cancer patients is 90 percent.[75] In 2016, researchers calculated that localized breast cancer, the form found in the majority of newly diagnosed cases, has a five-year survival rate of 99 percent.[76]

The National Cancer Institute biostatistician Robert Hoover once told his colleagues: "The scientific method I was taught involved setting a hypothesis and then trying everything you could to destroy it, and if you couldn't, then you began to accept it. Somehow we've gotten away from that. We develop hypotheses and then we do everything we can to find something that supports it."[77] That's not the way we should be doing science. Although we agree with Henry James's witty admission that "nothing is my last word on anything," we do think it is time to relegate the "common knowledge" that ERT and HRT cause breast cancer to the dustbin of discredited ideas—along with the theories that radical mastectomy is the best treatment for primary breast cancer, that anger causes peptic ulcers, and that stress causes tuberculosis.

2

The "Change of Life" and the Quality of Life

When Oprah Winfrey was forty-six years old, she developed attacks of severe heart palpitations. She saw at least five cardiologists, each of whom assured her that her heart was fine, but none of them could tell her what was causing the palpitations. She was frustrated, especially because, as she observed to her legions of fans, no physician would want to miss diagnosing her correctly since she was, in fact, Oprah Winfrey. She was still having regular periods and remained worried and annoyed by the palpitations until her trainer suggested that they could be a sign of early menopause.[1] *What?* Winfrey thought. *Menopause, at only forty-six?* But then she came upon a popular book, *The Wisdom of Menopause* by Dr. Christiane Northrup, that listed palpitations as a common symptom of menopause.

Heart palpitations certainly get a woman's attention, but other symptoms that are also signs of menopause usually do not, symptoms such as severe dryness of the eyes and mouth, which many women develop even when they are still having regular periods, or joint and muscle aches and pains. The list of symptoms associated with menopause includes other surprises as well as the familiar ones.

Hot flashes
Night sweats
Difficulty sleeping
Insomnia
Difficulty concentrating
Decreasing recent memory
Decreasing energy reserve
Bladder/urinary discomfort
More frequent urinary tract infections
Vaginal dryness
Vaginal discharge
Vaginal bleeding
Loss of sexual desire
Painful sexual intercourse
Depression/sadness
Tension/nervousness
Mood swings
Headaches
Bloating
Swelling of hands or feet
Breast tenderness
Aching joints

Thinning hair
Palpitations (racing heart)
Chest pain with exertion
Weight gain around the abdomen

That last entry is, of course, the lament of many women confronted with the dilemma of "Do I accept this change in waist size and get new clothes? Or do I wage war against the forces of biology and eat nothing but protein and work out three times a day?" People joke about "middle-aged spread" and usually attribute it to sloth, fast food, and too much sugar, but for women, menopause is also a major contributor. "I weigh the same as I always did," one of Av's patients grumbled, "but my fat cells seem to have redistributed themselves and reconvened in my belly."

The symptoms of menopause often begin in the years before periods stop completely (known as perimenopause) and can last for years afterward. But many women do not mention them to their doctors at all, let alone in any detail, sometimes because of shame or embarrassment, but often because, like Oprah Winfrey, they don't associate the problem with menopause. Heart palpitations send many women to cardiologists; aching muscles and joints send them to rheumatologists; insomnia sends them to sleep-disorder clinics; and depression sends them to psychotherapists or psychiatrists. One fifty-year-old woman we spoke to said, "I had suffered from insomnia for years, attributing it to work stresses and the kids. But once I started HRT, I slept soundly through the night for the first time in four years. The work is still stressful and the kids are still kids, but I sleep." A friend of Carol's said that when she entered menopause in her early fifties, she had none of the concerns her friends did—no hot flashes, no sleepless nights, no headaches—and so she didn't consider taking hormones. "Then, one night," she said, "I dreamed that I was happy—really happy—and when I awoke I realized I had not felt that joyful in too long. I didn't know that one symptom of menopause is depression. I called my doctor and began HRT right away, and I became my cheerful self again. I took it for years but stopped because she advised me to, after the WHI reports. I am still seething that I quit."

Echoing the complaints and concerns of many women in Av's practice, one psychotherapist wrote to us with her own observations:

> Every day in my practice I work with women who—either through their doctors' discouragement or due to their own fears and misinformation—have not taken estrogen and experienced its benefits. I see major depression and generalized anxiety disorder, ruined sexual and emotional connection with spouses, disintegrating marriages and fractured families as a result. Of course, the depletion of estrogen in menopause is not the single cause of these problems, but I'm certain it plays a predominant role in the abrupt loss of these women's (and their families') quality of life after menopause.

Oh, it does. In *The Madwoman in the Volvo: My Year of Raging Hormones,* Sandra Tsing Loh's hilarious account of her midlife crisis induced by menopause, the author describes the miseries of being "estrogen-deprived," many of which are funny (at least afterward, and at least when described by a professional humorist). There she is, pulling off the road to sob—"producing heaves of seawater like Jonah's whale"—about the death of her children's hamster: "I am a forty-nine-year-old woman sitting in her filthy Volvo parked under a tree on a Tuesday afternoon wailing about a hamster. Just how low are we setting the bar here?" (Though, she adds, it was an adorable hamster with a sunny disposition.) Her good friend Ann, hearing the story, gently suggests Loh might be entering menopause. But the fanatical regimen that Ann has adopted to deal with her depression and rage attacks—"a cocktail of antidepressants, bioidenticals, walks, facials, massages, dark chocolate, and practically throwing salt over her shoulder"—does not help Loh. Eventually, Loh finds salvation and sanity in putting topical estrogen cream on her wrists.[2]

Individual experiences are illuminating but they are not scientific evidence; for one thing, people are often famously incorrect about the causes of their physical and emotional concerns. For example, starting in their fifties, both sexes tend to gain weight. Many women are so hyperalert to their weight that they latch onto any culprit they can blame, but at least the ones who aren't taking hormones can rule out HRT. "There is a general belief among women and even some doctors that menopause hormones contribute to weight gain," wrote Tara Parker-Pope in *The Hormone Decision*. "The scientific data simply do not support this."[3] In a large, yearlong study that compared menopausal women on hormones with those who were on a placebo, most of the women gained some weight—but the hormone group gained less than the placebo group. And in the Women's Health Initiative, a higher proportion of those on HRT *lost* weight compared to the women on placebo.[4]

Likewise, depression, anxiety, marital unhappiness, and sexual problems occur for many different reasons—physiological, psychological, and troubles with Harold. But in this chapter, we will argue that the drop in estrogen is an underrecognized cause of the wide array of symptoms that emerge during menopause. We will consider the evidence showing why estrogen remains the most effective treatment for these symptoms, and we will evaluate the claims that bioidentical products or alternative therapies are just as effective as estrogen without the alleged risks. But first we want to acknowledge the historical, cultural, and political context of this contentious issue.

ESTROGEN: THE JEKYLL AND HYDE OF TREATMENTS

Over its long history, estrogen has been seen as everything from a cure-all for any and every female complaint to a dangerous, even disastrous drug; from a kindly Dr. Jekyll to a fiendish Mr. Hyde; from the solution to the problem. "The story of estrogen," Elizabeth Siegel Watkins wrote in *The Estrogen Elixir,* her fascinating history of HRT in America, "is woven from several strands: blind faith in the ability of science and technology to solve a broad range of health and social problems, social and cultural stigmatization of aging, shifting meanings and interpretations of femininity and female identity, and the pitfalls of medical hubris in the twentieth century."[5] Women wanting to make decisions about hormone replacement therapy struggle to untangle those strands. Is taking HRT antifeminist or profeminist? Why is *replacement* a bad word when it refers to menopause hormones but not a bad word when it refers to, say, replacing thyroid hormones if the thyroid gland is removed? (And given that, after menopause, estrogen drops to about 1 percent of the levels in premenopausal women, *replacement* seems precisely the right word.[6]) Does HRT medicalize a problem that would be better treated with psychotherapy or a new job? Is it healthier to tough it out and suffer in silence or try hormones?

The 1970s, with the birth of the modern feminist movement, saw a sharp split emerge among feminists on the subject of estrogen. The decade was off to a roaring start with *Our Bodies, Ourselves,* a book that was greeted with well-deserved fanfare in 1971; it urged women to learn about their bodies, health, and sexuality and take control of their own medical care. In 1977, two popular books anchored the feminist anti-estrogen position: Rosetta Reitz, a member of the New York Radical Feminists, published *Menopause: A Positive Approach,* and Barbara and Gideon Seaman published *Women and the Crisis in Sex Hormones.* As Watkins wrote, "These two books reflected the contemporary critical stance against the organized medical profession and the pharmaceutical industry and the concurrent fascination with so-called natural approaches to health care."[7] Those natural approaches, still recommended today, were exercise, calcium, "good nutrition" (however it was defined that year), and, for Reitz, perhaps telling us more about herself than the general population, having regular sex and healthy relationships. Both of these successful books regarded hormone therapy of any kind as either unnecessary or harmful. But their main strengths lay in their clarion call to women to resist the paternalism of the medical establishment and reject the insulting language of menopause as being a "deficiency disease" and the pervasive, sexist notion that once past menopause, women were, literally and figuratively, washed-up.

Yet the very success of feminism was sending more women into science, research, and medicine. In the same year that Reitz and the

Seamans published their books, Lila Nachtigall, an obstetrician-gynecologist at NYU who at the time was halfway through her own twenty-two-year research study, published *The Lila Nachtigall Report*. The book urged women to educate and thereby empower themselves, and it provided comprehensive information about menopause and the therapeutic benefits of estrogen. Nachtigall entered medical school in 1956, one of four women in her class, and had worked as an advocate for women ever since. But in the newly exuberant feminism of the 1970s, Watkins observed, "*The Lila Nachtigall Report* didn't stand a chance. Written by a doctor who was promoting the use of a drug that was at the nadir of its popularity, castigated by scientists and feminists alike, the book was out of step with the times."[8] Nine years later, in 1986, Nachtigall published *Estrogen: The Facts Can Change Your Life*. The climate had changed. The benefits of estrogen — in preventing osteoporosis, Nachtigall's specialty, and promoting heart health — were repeatedly demonstrated. Until, of course, the Women's Health Initiative set that pendulum swinging back again.

Today, many feminists and health activists continue to oppose HRT for social and political reasons as well as health concerns. After the Women's Health Initiative's press release in 2002, Cynthia Pearson, executive director of the National Women's Health Network, told Gina Kolata of the *New York Times* how pleased she was that the WHI had validated her opposition to HRT. The advocacy of HRT, she told Kolata, was "sexist and ageist, with its message that women should: Stay healthy. Stay sexually vital. Be less of a pain to your husband."[9]

Sexist and ageist, really? At a conference devoted to the treatment of estrogen-deficiency symptoms, Nachtigall noted: "Among

2,000 postmenopausal women in a given year, 20 will develop heart disease, 11 bone loss, 6 breast cancer, and 3 endometrial cancer, but nearly 100 percent will develop urogenital atrophy. Urogenital atrophy is not the first sign of menopause, but rather occurs gradually after the onset of the climacteric."[10] The symptoms include vaginal itching, urinary burning, urinary frequency, and painful sexual intercourse. Although not life-threatening, urogenital atrophy, if left untreated, will persist and worsen as a woman ages.

We are fully aware of the many women, and men, whose attitude toward sex in their later years is "free at last"; we do not wish to imply that everyone wants, or should want, to be sexually active. But we think it is just as misguided to assume that most women in their middle and late years do *not* want to be sexually active. To see the bias, reread that list of symptoms at the start of this chapter, omitting breast tenderness and vaginal discomfort, as if it applied to men. How would men respond to being told, "Buck up, guys! It's normal aging! Don't worry about those chest pains and bloating and headaches, the sleepless nights and memory lapses! No interest in sex anymore? Painful intercourse? Hey, you're over fifty; you've had enough sex already. Oh, your wife still enjoys sex? Too bad; be less of a pain to her about it. Besides, those symptoms will last only a few years, though more than half of you men will still have those symptoms for another decade or more, and some of you will have painful intercourse from now on. A lubricant will help if you want sex, but it won't help you want sex."

It would be hard to imagine most men accepting that message.

Of course, we know what Pearson meant by "ageist"—the ubiquitous cultural message that old is bad, young is good, and all of us, men and women alike, should fight signs of age with every weapon at hand. The non-ageist view held by many feminists is that the symptoms of menopause are as normal a part of life as menarche and therefore something to be tolerated, while repeating King Solomon: "This too shall pass." If symptoms are severe, they can be treated with alternatives to medication. In this view, menopause can be dealt with in the same way that people deal with any other sign of age, such as gray hair or wrinkles — try some over-the-counter aids or do nothing. A friend of ours, a college professor, hated having hot flashes and the resultant profusion of sweat that left her drenched, but she treated it all matter-of-factly, once telling her class: "This is what hot flashes look like. I'm not about to faint or die. Now hand in your papers."

Moreover, we share Pearson's and other consumer advocates' criticism of Big Pharma's unregulated ability to advertise directly to consumers, generate new medications by barely changing a molecule in older, effective ones, and expand markets for medications where none are needed. We too are sympathetic to the Less Is More movement, which is trying to educate the public so they will avoid unnecessary medications and diagnostic tests. We too condemn "disease-mongering," the arbitrary creation of new diseases, usually done by extending the borders of real medical conditions to include "pre-" conditions that do not and may never need medication. (As we will discuss in chapter 4, *osteopenia,* allegedly a precursor of osteoporosis, is one such manufactured term, propelled to its status, as one medical historian wrote, "by aggressive marketing and vested interests."[11])

We can't deny that estrogen too has had aggressive marketing and vested interests behind it, starting with Robert Wilson's *Femi-*

nine Forever and its claim that women can't be "fully female" without estrogen. In the years following that book's publication, many physicians handed out hormones readily and pressured their patients to take them and not ask pesky questions. Many physicians in those years were arrogant, sexist, and patriarchal, with menopause portrayed in medical textbooks as a "deficiency disease" or "ovarian failure."[12] No wonder that women who went through menopause in those decades tended to become skeptical of HRT; it was hard to separate the question of hormones from the condescension of the (mostly) men prescribing them. Carol's mother, Dorie, loved telling the story of what happened when her gynecologist asked when she had had her last period.

"Hmm," she'd said, reflecting. "It's been about a year, come to think of it."

"Are you having hot flashes, sleeplessness, aches, and pains?" he asked.

"No," she said, "though I did have a chill in a movie theater once."

"Here," he said, not listening, "have this prescription filled; it will help."

Years have gone by since that conversation, and the needle of estrogen advice has moved from pro to con. Today, we are convinced that having that prescription filled *will* often help, after all.

Menopause and Beyond

As far as we know, the only animal besides humans that goes through menopause and lives for many years thereafter is the whale, making this phenomenon something of an evolutionary mystery. (We have no information about what symptoms orca or pilot whales experience or whether eating herring eggs alleviates them.) The grandmother hypothesis holds that in ancient times, human infants and children were more likely to survive if their grandmothers were around to care for them and were not in sexual competition with their daughters for partners and resources.[13] But whatever the evolutionary reason for menopause, due to the extraordinary advances in health and sanitation in the past century, the great majority of modern women live an average of three decades after menopause, making the issue of improving their health and their quality of life more pressing.

Some women have virtually no symptoms during menopause; like Carol and her mother, their periods just stop, and that's that. But they are a minority. According to the Study of Women's Health Across the Nation (SWAN), a multiracial/multiethnic study that followed 3,302 women as they entered menopause between 1996 and 2013, about 80 percent of women experience some symptoms, and for half of them, those symptoms last for years. The median duration of hot flashes and other vasomotor symptoms among these women was 7.4 years; it was even longer (10 years) for African American women and upwards of 12 years for women whose symptoms began during perimenopause.[14]

The Women's Health Initiative did not even want to grant that HRT might help alleviate these unpleasant symptoms. The WHI reported in 2003 that estrogen did not have a "clinically meaningful effect on health-related quality of life," even among women who had taken it for three years.[15] When Av told his wife, Martha, this, she laughed out loud. She had been pushed into menopause at the age of forty-six as a result of chemotherapy and almost immediately developed hot flashes, night sweats, and difficulty sleeping. Within days of Martha's starting estrogen, those symptoms diminished and then disappeared. It usually takes less than a week for most symptomatic menopausal women to feel better after beginning HRT; how in the world did the WHI get such an anomalous result?

When their study began, the WHI researchers were not interested in the effect of hormones on menopausal symptoms; they were investigating the hormones' effects on the big problems, notably breast cancer, heart disease, and cognitive impairment. Then why did they publish an article on the menopausal symptoms they had not set out to study? We don't know, but it feels to us that they were reluctant to admit that HRT was beneficial to women for *anything*. We say this because the WHI researchers wrote that they explicitly discouraged women who reported having "moderate or severe" menopausal symptoms from participating. As a result, women who had moderate or severe symptoms made up only 13 percent of the study participants. (Recall that the median age of these women was sixty-three, so most of the symptoms they might have had at the onset of menopause and for the subsequent decade would have passed.) However, among those 13 percent with symptoms, more than three-fourths randomized to take HRT rather than placebo reported substantial relief—just as every other study has found. The rest of the sample, the women who had had either no symptoms or minimal symptoms, reported no relief of symptoms. Let's repeat that: *The women who didn't have symptoms reported that estrogen did not relieve the symptoms they didn't have.* And that is how the WHI got its "finding" that HRT did not have a "clinically meaningful effect on health-related quality of life"[16]—by focusing on the 87 percent who had had no symptoms at the outset and were way past menopause in any case. The authors themselves noted that their data "may not be applicable to [women with moderate to severe symptoms], because women who believed they needed hormone therapy were unlikely to agree to undergo randomization."

We are not making this up.

Another way the WHI could claim that HRT did not improve quality of life relied on how the investigators measured "quality of life." They didn't do it by offering participants a list of specific symptoms, as we did at the start of this chapter, and asking them to assess the severity of each one, ranging from "not at all troubling" to "tolerable" to "unbearable," and noting whether and how it was affecting their lives. Instead, they relied on vague assessments, asking participants to rate their well-being, mood, ways of coping, and general health. When people are asked for global evaluations like these, they typically respond as you probably do when an acquaintance asks you how you are. You most likely say, "Oh, I'm fine. All good." You don't mention the sweats, sleeplessness, palpitations, or, for that matter, your problems with Harold. (Similarly, on national opinion polls, when people are asked how happy they are overall, about two-thirds say "very happy." Ask them about particular aspects of their lives and you'll get the truth: "My shoulder pain has finally gone away but I'm super-stressed by my boss and ready to send my sullen teenager to boot camp.") Global assessments, in short, play off women's tendency to cope and not complain about particular symptoms that are interfering with work or family life.

But even the WHI could not overturn the medical consensus that estrogen is the most effective treatment for the symptoms that Martha and millions of other women have, eliminating or reducing them in the great majority of women who take HRT or ERT. "To this day," wrote Elizabeth Watkins in 2007, "estrogen remains the single most effective remedy for the hot flashes of menopause, and few critics dispute its value as a temporary treatment."[17] Multiple randomized trials reviewed by oncologist Heidi Nelson of the Mayo Clinic in 2004 found that estrogen generally reduces the frequency of hot flashes by more than 75 percent.[18] Guidelines from the American College of Obstetrics and Gynecology state that "because some women age 65 or more might still need HRT for vasomotor symptoms, HRT should not be routinely discontinued at age 65, but, as in younger women, should be individualized."[19] The North American Menopause Society concurs.

The WISDOM study, an acronym for the Women's International Study of Long-Duration Oestrogen After the Menopause, was a randomized, placebo-controlled trial of 3,721 postmenopausal women in Australia, New Zealand, and the United Kingdom. The women ranged in age from fifty to sixty-nine and were randomly assigned to take HRT or placebo. The study found that compared to the women given the placebo, those women on HRT experienced improved sleep, reduced hot flashes and night sweats, fewer aching joints and muscles, less vaginal dryness, and improved sexual functioning.[20] (The only negative side effects were that women on HRT were slightly more likely to report breast tenderness and vaginal discharge.) The researchers particularly emphasized the benefits of HRT on improving sleep and reducing insomnia, given that inadequate sleep is "associated with an increased risk of illnesses such as obesity, diabetes, hypertension, and cardiovascular disease. Reducing sleep deprivation might therefore have considerable health benefits."

Further, because many menopausal women report joint and muscle pain and increased arthritic symptoms—as we said, that's another set of symptoms not popularly associated with menopause—the WISDOM researchers highlighted their finding that women reported lower levels of bodily pain after a year on HRT. Indeed, they cited the WHI, which had (quietly) gotten the same result: "A follow-up study with participants in the Women's Health Initiative that looked at joint symptoms showed a higher prevalence of pain or stiffness in those women who stopped taking combined HRT compared with placebo."[21] Research on animals, they added, suggested that estrogen also "has an anaesthetic role and might prevent cartilage erosion such as occurs in osteoarthritis."[22]

Although the WISDOM study found no alleviation of symptoms of depression among the participants, other randomized trials of ERT have reported remarkable improvements in depression. Two randomized, placebo-controlled studies in which women suffering from depressive episodes received four to twelve weeks of estrogen or placebo found a 60 to 75 percent improvement in the estrogen group versus a 20 to 30 percent improvement for women given placebo.[23] That estrogen has such a high rate of success in lifting depression—much better than what research has found for antidepressants and without the often unpleasant side effects of antidepressants[24]—is tremendously important. Katie Taylor, an Englishwoman, was her own control group in experiencing the difference between antidepressants and HRT:

A few years ago, I was 43, and had just returned to work after a long break bringing up my four children. I loved my life, but was feeling exhausted, teary and down, for no obvious reason. My GP diagnosed depression and prescribed anti-depressants. This, it turned out, was a misdiagnosis. After six months, I felt worse. I had "brain fog," couldn't think clearly at work, cried at the most inconvenient moments, had hot flushes and didn't want to leave the house.... The anti-depressant turned me into a zombie, I felt nothing—it just wasn't right. I feared it was the pressure of combining home life with a demanding job.... I talked to my GP again and she agreed I should stop working and focus on my own health and looking after my family.[25]

That "stop working" was more bad advice, advice that many women can't afford to take. Fortunately for her, Katie Taylor is the daughter of Michael Baum, one of England's preeminent cancer researchers, and he suggested that, young as she was, she might be in menopause. And that was the right diagnosis; she was indeed. She began HRT, got off the antidepressant, "got the old Katie back" with her former cheerfulness and energy, and even started an online support group to provide information for women going through menopause.

For women who have survived breast cancer, chemotherapy typically induces menopause and intensifies its symptoms.[26] Dawn Hershman, leader of the Breast Cancer Program of the Herbert Irving Comprehensive Cancer Center at Columbia University, reported that women treated with chemotherapy were 5.7 times more likely to report vaginal dryness, 5.5 times more likely to report painful sexual intercourse, 3 times more likely to report decreased libido, and 7.1 times more likely to report difficulty achieving orgasm than women who didn't have chemo.[27] Between 66 and 96 percent of breast cancer survivors report having severe hot flashes, night sweats, and insomnia, and the great majority fail to receive treatment for these annoying and uncomfortable symptoms.[28]

Many cancer survivors are understandably preoccupied with coping with the effects of their illness and are relieved that its treatment is over, and because of their worry that estrogen might increase the risk of recurrence, they are inclined to endure menopausal symptoms as an inevitable side effect of chemotherapy. Yet in a 2017 review of observational and prospective randomized studies of breast cancer survivors titled "Use of Hormone Therapy for Menopausal Symptoms and Quality of Life in Breast Cancer Survivors: Safe and Ethical?," two gynecologists answered that question with an unqualified yes. In all of these cases, the authors, María Fernanda Garrido-Oyarzún (in Santiago, Chile) and Camil Castelo-Branco (in Barcelona, Spain) concluded that the best treatment was estrogen.[29] Av's own research supports that conclusion, as we will discuss fully in chapter 6.

Today, many gynecologists and oncologists still struggle to reconcile their suspicions that estrogen is dangerous and doesn't improve quality of life with the clear evidence of its benefits. Many have come up with a curious compromise: it is safe for *some* women with severe symptoms to take hormones if they do it for the briefest time and in the smallest dose possible. This advice represents a compromise between *It's dangerous—don't take it at all* and *It's safe—take it as long as you like.* Of course, if physicians really believe that estrogen is carcinogenic, they shouldn't advise taking it at all; that is like saying, "Smoke a half a pack of cigarettes a day, but only for a year, and you'll sleep better."

This is the bottom line: there is no scientific basis for the admonition to take as low a dose of postmenopausal hormones for as short a period as possible. According to the 2017 hormone-therapy position statement of the North American Menopause Society, "The concept of 'lowest dose for the shortest time' may be inadequate or even harmful for some women." And, its authors added, "there are no data to support routine discontinuation [of HRT] in women age 65 years."[30]

Ten years after their original paper, in a follow-up study published in 2012, the WHI finally admitted that estrogen did, in fact, significantly reduce vasomotor symptoms such as light-headedness, dizziness, and hot flashes and that those symptoms recurred as soon as the women stopped taking estrogen.[31] In fact, one of the principal investigators, JoAnn Manson, allowed that women could now safely take HRT without fear that it would cause early death: "This is good news for women," she told the *Times* (UK). "This fundamentally provides reassurance for women during the menopause who are seeking hormone therapy to manage bothersome and disturbing symptoms such as hot flushes and night sweats."[32] Three years later, in 2015, Manson and Gloria Richard-Davis of the University of Arkansas Medical Sciences wrote a commentary, "Research Overturns Dogma," on that large-scale SWAN study. In it, they commended the researchers for overturning "the dogma that [vasomotor symptoms] have a short duration, minimally affect women's health or quality of life and can be readily addressed by short-term approaches."[33]

They praised the overturning of the dogma that they themselves created? While we regret that Manson originally promoted the inappropriately alarmist interpretations of the WHI findings, not even recognizing HRT's benefits on menopausal symptoms, we are pleased that she has been able to change her mind—a little. "There was a lot of fear," she said, not quite admitting that it was primarily the WHI that generated that fear.

What About the Alternatives?

All drugs, from aspirin to Zyrtec, have potential side effects and risks, and HRT is no exception. With hormone replacement, side effects include dry eyes, vaginal discharge, and breast tenderness, all of which can continue in some women for as long as one year. HRT also has small but more serious risks, including gallbladder disease and blood clots in veins. (We will evaluate the balance of risks versus benefits in chapter 8.) Understandably, many women don't like taking prescription drugs unless it is medically necessary; others feel (thanks to the WHI) that HRT is riskier than other medication options. Let's consider them.

Some women may decide to do nothing and endure their discomforts. Those women who want to do something but don't want to take estrogen, with or without progesterone, have three choices: take prescription drugs for specific menopausal symptoms, try any of the zillions of botanicals and other "natural" products marketed for menopause, or get a prescription for a bioidentical version of estrogen. We won't even discuss the ever-popular all-purpose pabulum about "individualized lifestyle modifications and nonpharmacologic therapies" for treating symptoms, such as these recommendations from the *Journal of Clinical Endocrinology and Metabolism:* women should stop smoking, lose weight, drink less alcohol, take vitamin D and calcium, eat a healthy diet, use vaginal lubricants, and get regular physical activity. And for severe hot flashes and sleepless nights, the authors of the article added, cognitive behavioral therapy, hypnosis, and acupuncture "may be helpful."[34] All perfectly sensible advice (apart from taking vitamin D and calcium, which are mostly useless and have no benefit even for preventing fractures in postmenopausal women, as we will see in chapter 4), but unfortunately none of these approaches alleviates menopausal symptoms.

Some women are given the antiseizure medication gabapentin (Neurontin), a drug primarily used to treat seizures and nerve pain but increasingly used for off-label purposes such as treating hot flashes. Neurontin does help reduce hot flashes somewhat— though not as much as estrogen does[35]—but its side effects include (to list just a few) dizziness, drowsiness, fatigue, unsteadiness, nausea, diarrhea, constipation, headache, breast swelling, and dry mouth, and while it may reduce hot flashes, it doesn't help the other symptoms of menopause. In addition, it can cause seizures if stopped abruptly.

Antidepressants are widely prescribed and some studies have found them to be effective in reducing hot flashes and insomnia. One randomized, double-blind, placebo-controlled study of eighty women who had been treated for gynecological cancer found that patients given paroxetine (Paxil) had fewer hot flashes and nighttime awakenings.[36] But a larger review of the effectiveness of antidepressants concluded that "data on the benefits [of these medications] are conflicting."[37] And, of course, antidepressants come with their own often unpleasant side effects and risks and do not help women with any other symptoms. In 2013, an FDA panel rejected approval of gabapentin and paroxetine for hot flashes, noting that both drugs had only marginal benefit.[38]

By far the most widely used alternatives to HRT are botanicals and natural products like over-the-counter Chinese herbs, black cohosh, ginseng, Saint-John's-wort, and ginkgo biloba. Some physicians, even those who believe that HRT is safe for the majority of women, want to offer alternatives to women who don't want to take hormones; they often end up suggesting a cocktail of herbs, one for this symptom and another for that one. Physicians at the Well Woman Centre in Dublin, who regard HRT as the "most effective prescription medicine for menopause," suggest that women who don't want to take hormones might consider "Omega 3s for brain function, vitamin D for bones, Starflower Oil for breast tenderness. Vitamin E oil can be used for vaginal dryness."[39] Countless popular books of menopause advice recommend these herbal products, a multibillion-dollar industry, but study after study finds that none of them reduces menopausal symptoms any more than placebos do. A sampling:

— The Isoflavone Clover Extract Study, a randomized controlled trial of two dietary supplements derived from red clover extract (sold as Promensil and Rimostil), found that they did not differ from placebo in reducing hot flashes or improving menopausal quality of life.[40]

— Deborah Grady, professor of medicine and of epidemiology and biostatistics at the Women's Health Clinical Research Center at the University of California, San Francisco, concluded that numerous randomized trials have demonstrated that estrogen markedly diminishes the frequency and severity of hot flashes by 80 to 95 percent but that "there is no convincing evidence that acupuncture, yoga, Chinese herbs, dong quai, evening primrose oil, ginseng, kava, or red clover extract improve hot flushes."[41]

—A meta-analysis in *JAMA* of nonhormonal therapies for hot flashes found that most studies have been of poor quality, making generalizability of limited use. "Adverse effects and costs may restrict use for many women," the researchers concluded. "These therapies may be most useful for highly symptomatic women who cannot take estrogen but are not optimal choices for most women."[42]

—A randomized trial of alternative medicines for menopausal symptoms—black cohosh, multibotanicals, and soy—compared with hormone therapy and placebo found no meaningful reduction in the number or intensity of symptoms in the women taking herbal supplements or placebo. Hormone therapy, however, significantly reduced symptoms.[43]

—A double-blind, randomized, placebo-controlled crossover trial of black cohosh in the management of hot flashes, published in the *Journal of Clinical Oncology*, "failed to provide any evidence that black cohosh reduced hot flashes more than the placebo."[44]

—A randomized controlled trial of acupuncture for treating hot flashes in breast cancer patients found no statistical difference between acupuncture and sham acupuncture.[45] (In sham-acupuncture studies, the needles are blunted and do not penetrate the skin or they're randomly inserted at places where theoretically they would have no benefit.)

We could keep going, but you get the picture: Repeatedly, double-blind studies find that about 20 percent of women who take herbs—red clover, soy, flaxseed, dong quai, evening primrose oil, ginseng, wild yam, chaste tree, hops, and sage—report improvement of symptoms, precisely the percentage among women given the placebo. (We don't even know what chaste tree is, but we are pleased that someone studied it.) One review, after concluding that claims about the efficacy and safety of herbs for menopause symptoms were largely unproved, warned about a possible association between black cohosh and liver toxicity.[46] That is why the American College of Obstetrics and Gynecology's practice guidelines explicitly note that complementary botanicals and natural products, including over-the-counter isoflavones, Chinese herbs, black cohosh, ginseng, Saint-John's-wort, and ginkgo biloba, have not been shown to be effective. Save your money.

Finally, let us consider bioidenticals. A typical endorsement turned up in "The Truth About Hormone Therapy," an op-ed in the *Wall Street Journal* written by three physicians—Erika Schwartz, Kent Holtorf, and David Brownstein. The essay began with an uncritical acceptance of the WHI's findings, claiming that "hormone-replacement therapy has become a textbook example of how special interests, a confused medical establishment, and opportunists can combine to complicate the issue and deny patients access to safe and effective treatments."[47] Fortunately, the authors said, the Women's Health Initiative brought HRT to "an abrupt halt" because it "proved unequivocally that the drugs were *unsafe* and significant factors in increasing the risk of heart attacks, strokes and breast cancer in the more than 16,000 women studied." What was a woman to do? Women were feeling horrible as they went off HRT, and their physicians, hostages to the medical establishment, had nothing to offer except antidepressants. Don't worry! Bioidentical drugs to the rescue! They are identical, so they work, but not exactly identical, so they aren't harmful. Drs. Schwartz, Holtorf, and Brownstein are founding members of the Bioidentical Hormone Initiative.

How can a drug be identical but not the same? *Bioidentical* is a marketing term, and quite a brilliant one at that, because it implies that it provides all the benefits of estrogen without... what? Estrogen's risks? Bioidenticals, which require a prescription just as HRT does, usually contain estradiol, the predominant form of circulating estrogen in women.* Premarin contains at least ten forms of estrogen, including estradiol, but it also has equilin, the form believed to be most beneficial in preserving brain function.[48] Nonetheless, commercially manufactured estrogen and bioidentical estrogen (usually estradiol) are approved and regulated by the FDA.

In contrast, *compounded* bioidentical hormones, which are widely used in the United States, are generally prepared by a local pharmacy according to a prescription written by a woman's physician. They are not standardized pharmaceutical products, they are not regulated by the FDA, and all major medical societies have discouraged their use as an alternative to approved forms of estrogen and progesterone.[49] Why, then, are they popular? An informal focus group of twenty-one women who were using or had used compounded bioidenticals were asked about their reasons for avoiding conventional HRT. They mentioned fear of its risks, an aversion to "mares' urine," and, most of all, an "overarching distrust of a medical system perceived as dismissive of their concerns and

---

* Estradiol is found in yams, but don't even think about it. You'd have to eat a *lot* of yams.

overly reliant on pharmaceuticals." They also enjoyed what they regarded as the "enhanced clinical care and attention" they got from their alternative-care doctors. "We find," the researchers concluded, "that women are not only seeking alternatives to conventional pharmaceuticals, but alternatives to conventional care where their menopausal experience is solicited, their treatment goals are heard, and they are engaged as agents in managing their own menopause."[50] It seems an unfortunate trade-off—to get the kind of physician who will listen, explain, and collaborate with them, they choose risky or ineffective treatments.*

As with all over-the-counter herbs and potions, consumers need to be aware of sciencey-sounding interventions that have no scientific basis, even when the advice comes from physicians who claim to be specialists in treating menopause. One such physician wrote to Avrum and commended him for his critique of the Women's Health Initiative but added that she nonetheless still opposed HRT. She herself, she said, preferred "bioidentical hormone replacement therapy (BHRT) and the Wiley Protocol," claiming they had better safety and efficacy than conventional HRT. When Av asked her for studies demonstrating that overall "safety and efficacy," she did not respond.

---

* The price of choosing an alternative medicine because it sounds or feels good can be high. In 2018, the *Journal of the National Cancer Institute* reported a study of death rates from *nonmetastatic* cancer over a five-and-a-half-year window. The researchers compared outcomes for 280 patients who chose alternative medicine instead of chemotherapy, radiotherapy, and surgery, with 560 patients treated traditionally. The patients who relied on unproven alternatives were, on average, 2.5 times more likely to die within that time, and for some cancers, the risk associated with alternative medicine was much worse: almost six times higher for patients with breast cancer and four times higher for colon cancer. (Johnson SB, Park HS, Gross CP, Yu JB. Use of alternative medicine for cancer and its impact on survival. JNCI. 2018;110:121–24.)

The Wiley Protocol is a bioidentical hormone system devised by Teresa S. Wiley, who has no scientific or medical credentials. Wiley claims that her method not only alleviates menopausal symptoms but also increases overall health and, who knows, may make you rich while you sleep.[51] We can't improve on Wikipedia's summary: "The protocol has been criticized by members of the medical community for the dosages of the hormones used, side effects of the treatment, potential physiologic effects, Wiley's lack of medical or clinical qualifications to design the protocol, lack of empirical evidence demonstrating it as safe or effective, ethical problems with the clinical trial that is being run to test it and potential financial conflicts of interest regarding financial incentives." Is that all?

The Take-Home

While we agree with the feminist critique of the overmedicalization of women's everyday life problems, we also believe the solution is not to undermedicalize them, either, and ignore or incorrectly treat symptoms and problems that have clear physiological origins. The goal, surely, is what is best for an individual woman. For Katie Taylor, the solution was neither antidepressants nor quitting her demanding job; it was taking hormones. Often, after Avrum's patients begin HRT, they call him, very upset. "I had felt old and used up," one woman said, "but after being on estrogen, the self I thought was long gone was back. I'm angry at all the time I wasted feeling miserable."

If HRT were of benefit only for women like this patient, that would be reason enough to endorse it. Indeed, as we have seen, the pendulum has begun to swing back to an acceptance of the evidence that HRT is beneficial, with very low risks, for treating the most severe symptoms of menopause. Now the debate has moved to the next level: If a woman has no worrisome symptoms in menopause or had them but they have subsided over time, should she consider taking HRT to prevent future diseases and difficulties? For JoAnn Manson of the WHI, the answer is still no. The decline in the use of HRT that followed the WHI's original reports "was not optimal," she now says, because women were suffering from symptoms that disrupted sleep and impaired their quality of life, which in turn affected health. However, she added, "this does not mean that we're going back to 25 years ago where hormone therapy was used for prevention of cardiovascular disease."[52]

In the next chapter we will evaluate that statement. We know that many women would rather endure uncomfortable symptoms for a while than take something that might help them briefly but harm them in the long run. However, it now appears that HRT does more than just improve the quality of women's lives; it also saves lives and prolongs lives—as we are about to see.

3

Matters of the Heart

M y gynecologist is against estrogen not because of breast cancer risk," a woman wrote to Avrum, "but because of the perceived increased risk of heart disease. She thinks that statins are much safer than hormones. Is this true?"

Although breast cancer is the most common cancer affecting women in this country, lung cancer kills more women than breast cancer does, and both pale next to heart disease, which is the leading cause of death in American women. The American Cancer Society estimated that in 2018, about 266,110 women would develop breast cancer; 40,920 would die of breast cancer; and approximately 90 percent of the women diagnosed with breast cancer would be cured following initial treatment. In spite of that heartening statistic, breast cancer generates more anxiety than heart disease, even though the number of American women who die annually of heart disease—projected to be 298,840 in 2018—is more than seven times the number projected to die of breast cancer.[1]

Some people have suggested that women fear breast cancer more than heart disease because breast cancer affects women at a younger age than heart disease does. However, that belief is wrong; in every decade over age forty, more women die of heart disease than of breast cancer. Take a look at this table of causes of death among women in 2014, the last year for which numbers are available:

	Age 20–39	Age 40–59	Age 60–79	Age 80 and Over
Heart Disease	2,459	22,465	76,242	187,680
Breast Cancer	1,051	10,708	18,461	10,991

Surprising, isn't it? Heart disease kills more than twice as many women as breast cancer does, even young women under the age of forty, and it kills four times as many women between the ages of sixty and seventy-nine. This difference has been the case for decades. A 1997 editorial in the *Lancet* described a survey commissioned by the National Council on Aging of one thousand women between the ages of forty-five and sixty-four. The survey found that "61% said that the disease they most feared was cancer—predominantly breast cancer. By contrast, only 9% said that the condition they most feared was the disease most likely to kill them—heart disease." The editorial added, "These findings are almost identical to a survey released also in 1997 by the American Heart Association. Only 8% of women recognized that heart disease and stroke were their leading causes of death, responsible for the deaths of more women each year than the next 16 causes of death combined—including diabetes, all forms of cancer,

AIDS, and accidents."[2] (We will discuss the issue of stroke in chapter 5.)

In spite of its unmistakable risk to women, heart disease remains almost invisible to them. Women often say to us, "But I know so many women who have had breast cancer, and so few who have had heart problems!" One reason may be, as we now know, that symptoms of heart disease, congestive heart failure, and heart attacks in women often differ from those in men; the familiar heart-attack symptom of crushing pain in the chest and left arm is more common in men than women, and the primary signs in women are usually unrelated to chest pain. (They include discomfort in the neck, jaw, shoulder, upper back, or stomach, shortness of breath, pain in one or both arms, nausea, sweating, dizziness, and extreme or unusual fatigue, all of which can indicate many different problems.) Unlike in men, atherosclerotic disease in women may be hard to confirm. Many women who go to their doctors or the ER with acute coronary syndromes are found to have angiograms that are normal, demonstrating no obstructive coronary artery disease.[3]

In her book *Women Are Not Small Men,* Nieca Goldberg, head of the Women's Heart Health Program at Lenox Hill Hospital in New York, describes the different ways that the sexes experience heart disease, which will kill one of every two women. It is a message that women cardiologists have been trying to convey for decades, though one often drowned out in the pink-ribbon campaigns about breast cancer. (The American Heart Association has come up with its own campaign, Go Red for Women.) New York internist Marianne Legato founded and became director of the

Partnership for Gender-Specific Medicine at Columbia University precisely because of the emerging evidence that studies based on the "normal" (white) man in medicine did not invariably apply to women or to other ethnicities—and heart disease was one area in particular where the sexes differed. In her groundbreaking 1991 book, *The Female Heart,* Legato touted the benefits of estrogen in reducing the risks of heart disease.[4]

Another reason that women underestimate the risk of death from heart disease may stem from what cognitive psychologists call the "availability heuristic," the tendency to judge the probability of an event by how easy it is to think of instances of it and how emotionally compelling those instances are. Catastrophes and shocking accidents evoke a strong emotional reaction and thus stand out in our minds, becoming more "available" mentally than other kinds of negative events. This is why people overestimate the frequency of deaths from tornadoes and underestimate the frequency of deaths from asthma, which occur dozens of times more often than tornado deaths but do not make headlines, and why women overestimate the frequency of deaths from breast cancer—already so scary—and underestimate the frequency of deaths from heart disease. Years ago, when many people in Europe and America were in a panic about "mad cow disease," which affects the brain and can be contracted by eating meat from contaminated cows, researchers did a creative field study in France. Whenever newspaper articles reported the dangers of mad cow disease, beef consumption fell during the following month. But when news articles reported the same dangers but used the technical names of the disease—Creutzfeldt-Jakob disease and bovine spongiform encephalopathy—beef consumption stayed the same.[5] The more vivid label caused people to react emotionally and overestimate the danger. During the entire period of the supposed crisis, only six people in France were diagnosed with the disease, but an image of a mad cow—that sweet, placid creature running amok—is highly "available."

We suspect that breast cancer is more available mentally than the more vague and diverse symptoms of heart disease. Indeed, people are so attuned to the politics and fund-raising efforts surrounding breast cancer that when a female celebrity is diagnosed with it, she almost invariably goes public. Although never diagnosed with breast cancer herself, Angelina Jolie released the news that she had the BRCA gene, an inherited genetic predisposition to develop breast cancer, and had chosen to have a double mastectomy. Such revelations are seen as brave acts to raise public awareness—which of course they do. Indeed, as we were writing this chapter, our phones beeped with the breaking news that Julia Louis-Dreyfus had breast cancer, which she revealed on Instagram and Twitter. Although no details of her diagnosis were included, the world reacted as if she had announced her imminent death. "Our love and support go out to Julia and her family at this time," HBO said in a solemn statement to the *Los Angeles Times*. Meanwhile, Miley Cyrus did not send out tweets when she learned that she suffers from an intermittent elevated heart rate (tachycardia), though she freely discusses it when asked, and there were no public revelations about the heart attacks of Olivia Newton-John, Elizabeth Taylor, Lena Horne, Toni Braxton, Greer Garson, Barbara Stanwyck, Barbara Walters, Rosie O'Donnell, Star Jones...

Even women who have had breast cancer are more likely to die from heart disease than from breast cancer. Jennifer Patnaik, an epidemiologist at the Colorado School of Public Health, and her colleagues studied a population of 63,566 women diagnosed with breast cancer at the age of sixty-six or older, following them for an average of nine years. They found that heart disease was responsible for more deaths among this large population than breast cancer. "Attention to reducing the risk of cardiovascular disease," the researchers concluded, "should be a priority for the long-term care of women following the diagnosis and treatment of breast cancer."[6]

Today this is an accepted recommendation among oncologists. At the 2017 San Antonio Breast Cancer Symposium, Anne H. Blaes, a medical oncologist at the University of Minnesota's medical school, presented a paper showing that nonchemotherapy drugs classified as SERMs (selective estrogen-receptor modulators), often given to postmenopausal breast cancer survivors after their primary treatment, have the potential to damage cells that line the coronary arteries. Because these drugs are generally prescribed for women with no residual evidence of breast cancer, because many of these women will never develop another breast cancer, and because the drugs are usually administered for a minimum of five years, Blaes cautioned that SERMs may do more harm than good because "most women with breast cancer are at greater risk of dying from cardiovascular disease than from breast cancer."[7] In 2018, the American Heart Association, in its first official scientific statement on cardiovascular disease and breast cancer, concurred.[8]

DOES HRT HARM THE HEART? HOW WOULD WE KNOW?

Research on estrogen and heart disease has a very long history. Because the risk of heart disease rises after menopause,[9] many studies have sought to determine whether estrogen has significant cardiovascular benefits. Compelling evidence suggests that it does.

—Elizabeth Barrett-Connor, professor of preventive medicine at the University of California, San Diego, and principal investigator of the Postmenopausal Estrogen/Progestin Interventions trial (PEPI), and Trudy Bush, an epidemiologist at Johns Hopkins, reviewed the existing studies and concluded that "most, but not all, studies of hormone replacement therapy in postmenopausal women show around a 50% reduction in the risk of a coronary event in women using unopposed oral estrogen."[10] Their own study of nearly nine hundred women found that estrogen plus progestin was actually better than estrogen alone in reducing the risk of heart attacks.

—In 1991, cardiologist Lee Goldman and statistician Anna Tosteson, both then at Harvard Medical School, wrote a lead editorial for the *New England Journal of Medicine* titled "Uncertainty About Postmenopausal Estrogen: Time for Action, Not Debate." A consensus of epidemiological studies, they wrote, had shown that women who were given postmenopausal estrogen had a 40 to 50 percent reduction in the risk of coronary artery disease compared with women who had not taken hormones.[11]

—In 2000, Francine Grodstein, an epidemiologist at the Harvard School of Public Health and a lead investigator on the Nurses' Health Study, reported that estrogen reduced the development of primary cardiovascular disease by nearly 40 percent.[12]

—In two separate studies, researchers reported that women who had their ovaries removed had an increased risk of coronary heart disease, a risk that was minimized if they were taking estrogen.[13]

Some scientific investigators have quarreled with the validity of these studies, which are among the most respected observational studies in the medical literature, precisely because they are observational and not randomized controlled trials (RCTs).

We want to take a moment to explain their concerns and where we think they're wrong.

As we have noted, RCTs are considered the ideal method of conducting medical research; in an RCT, women are randomly assigned to receive hormones (or any other treatment whose effectiveness is being tested) or a placebo, and, when the study is double-blind, neither they nor the investigators know who is taking what. However, observational studies have several advantages over randomized controlled trials: they are less expensive, can be done more quickly, can include a broader range of patients, and can be conducted when an RCT would be impossible or unethical. In observational studies, participants are not randomly assigned to a treatment group or a control group; they are simply observed over time to see whether the intervention helped, harmed, or did nothing, compared with a similar group who received a placebo or no treatment at all. The main problem with this method is that if women can *choose* whether to take hormones or not instead of being randomly assigned to hormones or a placebo, they may be different in ways that influence the outcome. Perhaps healthier, wealthier, more educated women choose to take hormones, and it's their health, wealth, and education that are responsible for any health benefits, not the medication.

In the 1970s and 1980s, researchers who were comparing RCTs with observational studies identified another crucial problem: earlier observational studies tended to inflate positive treatment effects. One analysis showed that more than half of the observational trials of a particular treatment found that it was effective, but only 30 percent of the double-blind, randomized controlled trials did.[14] Understandably, many researchers concluded that observational studies should not be used at all for evidence-based medical care. "If you find that [a] study was not randomized," said the authors of a 1997 book on evidence-based medicine, "we'd suggest that you stop reading it and go on to the next article."[15]

If that were so, you'd have to stop reading this book and go on to the next one, because you would be wary of the observational studies we cite that have demonstrated the benefits of estrogen on reducing the risks of heart disease and other medical problems. However, while RCTs get respect, they are not without pitfalls. Not only do some have their own biases and statistical distortions — the Women's Health Initiative being the largest and most unfortunate example — but several reports have found that carefully conducted observational studies and randomized controlled trials usually produce similar results.[16]

According to a review of this issue in the *New England Journal of Medicine* by physicians Kjell Benson and Arthur Hartz, older comparisons of the two approaches were based on studies conducted in the 1960s and 1970s, but research since then has improved. Observational studies conducted between 1985 and 1998, Benson and Hartz found, were "methodologically superior to earlier studies... [including] a more sophisticated choice of data sets and better statistical methods" that may have eliminated some systematic bias. They were able to compare RCTs and observational studies for nineteen varied medical treatments and found that "the effects of treatment in observational studies and in randomized controlled trials were similar in most areas."[17] And when other researchers scoured leading medical journals to see which medical practices had stood the test of time, comparing findings from both methods twenty years after their publication, the conclusions were still valid in 87 percent of nonrandomized observational studies and in 85 percent of randomized trials.[18]

Even Sir Austin Bradford Hill, the distinguished medical statistician and epidemiologist at Britain's Medical Research Council—the man who developed and promoted the randomized controlled trial in medicine—came to believe it had all gone too far. "Two decades after introducing the randomized controlled trial," wrote psychiatrist David Healy, "having spent years waiting for the pendulum to swing from the personal experience of physicians to some consideration of evidence on a large scale, Austin Bradford Hill suggested that if such trials ever became the only method of assessing treatments, not only would the pendulum have swung too far, it would have come off its hook."[19]

So let's take a look now at what the WHI found about hormones' effects on heart disease. Contradicting the decades of evidence that preceded them, the study's researchers produced a murky set of conflicting papers. In 2002, the first year that the WHI published its results, cardiologist Jacques Rossouw, then principal investigator of the Women's Health Initiative, and his colleagues reported that women on HRT, but not those on ERT, had a slightly increased relative risk of "heart events," including angina, indications for bypass surgery or angioplasty, and death due to heart disease.[20] But this increased risk occurred only among women in the first year of taking HRT. In 2004, Leon Speroff, then professor of obstetrics and gynecology and director of the Women's Health Research Unit of the School of Medicine at Oregon Health Sciences University, independently reanalyzed the WHI data and reported that the increased risk of cardiac events was seen only among women who were twenty or more years beyond menopause at the time they joined the study.[21]

In 2007, Rossouw and his fellow investigators revised their findings, now concluding that women who started HRT within ten years of the onset of menopause actually *reduced* their risk of coronary artery disease, while those who started after that slightly increased their risk.[22] The (observational) Nurses' Health Study came to the same conclusion.[23] And then two RCTs likewise demonstrated the benefits of estrogen on heart disease.

— Shelley Salpeter, a geriatrics specialist and internist in San Mateo, California, and her colleagues conducted a meta-analysis of twenty-three randomized controlled trials with a total of 39,049 women. They found a 30 percent decreased incidence of heart attacks and cardiac deaths among young postmenopausal women treated with estrogen alone or with HRT.[24]

— A Danish team of endocrinologists and epidemiologists, led by Louise Schierbeck, randomized 1,006 healthy, recently post-menopausal women to receive either ERT (if they had had hysterectomies) or HRT (if they had not) or nothing. In 2002, after ten years of follow-up, those who were taking ERT or HRT had a 50 percent reduction in the incidence of acute cardiac events without any associated increase in the risk of cancer, venous thrombosis, or stroke.[25]

The reason for the WHI's contradictory findings about hormones and heart disease is almost certainly that the study was not based, as they claimed, on a sample of healthy women in their late forties and early fifties who were just entering menopause. On the contrary, as we have noted repeatedly, not only was the median age of the women in their sample sixty-three, but fully 70 percent were seriously overweight and half were obese. Nearly 50 percent were either current or past cigarette smokers and more than 35 percent had been treated for high blood pressure. Only 10 percent of the women were between fifty and fifty-four years old, and 70 percent were sixty to seventy-nine, an age range where we would expect to find previously formed atherosclerotic plaques. This means that atherosclerosis was probably present in the WHI population when the study began, yet women with these well-established risk factors for heart disease were not excluded from the analysis of the effects of hormones on cardiovascular events.[26]

The WHI investigators have repeatedly stated that all of the women they recruited were healthy and that in fact this was a prerequisite for participation in this study. But these assertions are difficult to reconcile with the medical histories of so many of their participants. Indeed, Bhagu Bhavnani at the University of Toronto and Ronald Strickler at the Henry Ford Hospital in Detroit concluded that "strong basic science and clinical observational evidence show a benefit of menopausal [hormone therapy] in the cardiovascular and central nervous systems. Data from recent RCTs [that is, the Women's Health Initiative] that included predominantly overweight women aged between 63 and 71 years have been reported to show more harm than benefit; the rush to generalize these studies to all women and all menopausal HT regimens is unjustified."[27]

In *Making Sense of Science,* Cornelia Dean, a science writer for the *New York Times,* dismissed the findings of the WHI as concisely as the little boy who announced that the emperor was naked:

"The study enrolled women whose mean age was 63. In other words, they had been a decade or more past menopause. What the study demonstrated, it seemed, was that starting replacement therapy ten years after menopause offered little benefit."[28]

In light of the studies demonstrating a beneficial effect of hormones among women with no indication of heart disease, some researchers have wondered whether hormones would benefit women with already narrowed coronary arteries and proven evidence of heart disease. In 1998, a large randomized study—the Heart and Estrogen/Progestin Replacement Study (HERS)—was set up to answer that question. It found a statistically significant increase in heart events in women with known coronary artery disease prior to receiving HRT—but only during the first year of use.[29]

Why should HRT increase cardiovascular risk only in the first year of use and only among older women? Scientists have known for years that the elasticity of the coronary arteries decreases after menopause, and studies of primates show that continuous estrogen keeps blood vessels healthy. They have also shown that administering estrogen after an interval of some years cannot reverse vascular damage.[30] These findings have been replicated in humans too, for example in the Estrogen Prevention of Atherosclerosis Trial (EPAT) in 2000 and in the Estrogen Replacement and Atherosclerosis (ERA) study in 2001.[31] One leading explanation of the first-year-risk finding is that among women who do not have heart disease, estrogen causes blood vessels to dilate (widen), thereby increasing the blood supply to the heart muscle. However, in women who *do* have underlying heart disease, estrogen can potentially be harmful, because it can induce inflammation in existing arterial plaques, causing a stable plaque to rupture, and can also promote bleeding into the plaque, both of which can lead to blockage of a critical coronary artery. Estrogen, with or without progesterone, may also cause platelet clumping, which can further obstruct an already compromised coronary artery. After the first year of hormone therapy, the increased risk is no longer apparent even in women with preexisting coronary artery disease. This analysis would explain why studies that have enrolled younger women, like the Nurses' Health Study, have found that HRT has a protective effect: younger women are less likely to have arterial plaques.

This conclusion was supported in a randomized controlled trial in which 643 healthy postmenopausal women were divided according to time since menopause (under six years or more than ten years) and randomly assigned to receive either HRT or placebo. Every six months for an average of five years, the investigators measured the thickness of the women's carotid arteries—an indication of potential cardiovascular problems—and assessed the existence and degree of atherosclerosis with CT scans. HRT was responsible for a significantly slower progression of atherosclerosis as compared to placebo, but only when it was begun within six years of menopause. There was no benefit when it was initiated ten or more years after menopause.[32]

After those "estrogen causes breast cancer" reports from the WHI in 2002, between 50 and 70 percent of women who had been taking estrogen or HRT went off hormone therapy completely.[33] Over the next decade, drawing on the information we have presented here, cardiologists and epidemiologists began raising concerns that the human cost of that decision was an increase in coronary artery disease and death from heart disease. A team of Finnish researchers led by Tomi Mikkola at Helsinki University followed 332,202 Finnish women over time to determine any health consequences of discontinuing HRT. They found a 26 percent (statistically significant) increased risk of cardiac death during the first year of going off HRT compared with all women, on hormones or not, and they found more than double the increased risk among those who stopped HRT (364 deaths) compared with those who continued (155 deaths).[34] This finding does not mean that HRT is detrimental; it suggests that when women go off HRT, the benefit to their vascular health dissipates and their risk of heart disease becomes the same as it would have been had they never taken hormones.

WHAT ABOUT THE ALTERNATIVES?

The logical question that follows from all of this research is: What should a woman do? Most physicians feel there is no reason for women to take hormones *primarily* to help forestall or prevent cardiovascular disease, given, they say, that alternatives for reducing the risk of heart disease are readily available. What are those alternatives? How effective are they?

"If you're going to use something to prevent atherosclerosis, your choice is statins, not hormones," said Jacques Rossouw, the WHI cardiologist.[35] Indeed, statins are the leading medications used to prevent atherosclerosis-related cardiac deaths in this country; they are among the most widely prescribed pills in the world. Statins, such as Lipitor and Zocor, are designed to reduce high serum cholesterol, although definitions of *high* began to change when statins were developed and marketed. High cholesterol was once 240, then 220, then 210.... At first, there was so much enthusiasm about statins that physicians were advised to prescribe them for almost all patients in middle age, even those with no symptoms or personal history of heart disease. (In 2008, there was a brief flurry of debate over proposed guidelines from the American Academy of Pediatrics to prescribe them for very young children with cholesterol levels above 200.[36]) The excitement about the benefits of statins drowned out concerns over their known side effects, which are not trivial; they include liver enzyme abnormalities, muscle weakness, joint pain, and diabetes[37]—none of which are side effects of estrogen.

To assess the value of statins, therefore, a woman at risk of heart disease needs to know two things: (1) Is high cholesterol on its own a significant risk factor; and (2) Do statins, in lowering cholesterol, lower that risk? The answers are no and no.

In *The Truth About Statins,* cardiologist Barbara H. Roberts, director of the Women's Cardiac Center at the Miriam Hospital in Providence, Rhode Island, reports that statins are less effective in women than men, that they have their greatest benefit in preventing a second heart attack, and that they are more of a marketing success story than a medical one.[38] In a major review supporting that conclusion, physicians Judith Walsh and Michael Pignone found thirteen studies of the effects of statins on women and men with and without cardiovascular disease. Six of these studies, representing 11,435 women *without* cardiovascular disease, showed that lowering cholesterol levels did not reduce overall mortality rates and did not lower the chances of having a nonfatal heart attack or other coronary heart disease problems. Eight studies representing

8,272 women who already had cardiovascular disease showed that statins did reduce the risk of nonfatal and fatal heart attacks.[39]

Furthermore — and this finding always comes as a shock to people — there is no relationship between total cholesterol level and death from heart disease, especially for women.[40] (We are not talking about subtypes of cholesterol, like LDL, or triglycerides, high levels of which are risk factors. But people tend to use the overall total as the danger sign, with 200 as the magic number to get under.) The long-running Framingham Heart Study discovered this in the mid-1970s,[41] and there's been no modification of that finding since, but few paid any attention. Twenty years later, cardiologist and health-care researcher Harlan Krumholz, at the Yale School of Medicine, and his colleagues reported no correlation between cholesterol levels and heart disease, especially in women and men over age seventy.[42] Few paid serious attention to their research either.

Well, then, how about just cutting out fat, that stuff that makes us fat and clogs our arteries and causes heart disease? In *Good Calories, Bad Calories,* the investigative journalist Gary Taubes presents an exhaustive history of how cholesterol and fat became the leading villains in the American diet.[43] The belief that fat is the bad guy was obvious, intuitive, widely promulgated, institutionalized in medical guidelines, and eventually shown to be wrong. It's not only wrong; it's really wrong. Fat isn't always a culprit, and often it's a benefactor. Consider the fascinating 2017 findings from the Prospective Urban Rural Epidemiology (PURE) project, which followed individuals age thirty-five to seventy in eighteen countries for about seven years.[44] The international team of investigators led by Mahshid Dehghan of the Population Health Research Institute at McMaster University kept meticulous dietary records of all 135,335 participants and later assessed their overall mortality and major cardiovascular events (fatal cardiovascular disease, nonfatal myocardial infarction, stroke, and heart failure). And this is what they found:

- Intake of total fat and each type of fat (saturated, mono-unsaturated, etc.) was associated with a *lower* risk of total mortality.
- Higher saturated fat intake was associated with a *lower* risk of stroke.
- Total fat and saturated and unsaturated fats were not associated with risk of myocardial infarction or death from cardiovascular disease.
- Higher carbohydrate intake was associated with a *higher* risk of total mortality.

Ain't science grand? And annoying, of course, because it tells us to change our minds when the weight of the evidence demands.

The Take-Home

When it comes to the issue of estrogen and heart disease, the basic questions are these: How do the risks and benefits of hormones balance out, and what evidence should women and their physicians trust to help them make decisions?

First, we can consider the findings from randomized controlled studies and observational studies, which have converged. As Howard Hodis, head of the Atherosclerosis Research Unit at the University of Southern California, told *Bioscience Technology* in 2015, "The data looked this good 13 years ago. The negative shadow [was due to the] way the data was spun [by the WHI]. But it is reassuring that the effects of hormone therapy (HT) still look so good. Hormone therapy *as studied by the WHI and observational studies all show that it reduces overall mortality* when initiated in young women in close proximity to menopause [emphasis ours]. In fact, data currently being published show that when women stop HT, death rates increase."[45] And the biggest contributor to those death rates is cardiovascular disease. HRT, Hodis and his colleagues concluded, when begun before age sixty or within ten years of entering menopause, significantly reduces coronary artery disease *and* overall mortality. Moreover, statins and aspirin do not have these beneficial effects. Statins and aspirin, they noted, have "not been conclusively shown to significantly reduce CHD [coronary heart disease]," and there is no evidence that either "reduces overall mortality in women."[46]

Next, we can turn to decision analysis, a method designed to help patients make personal medical decisions that reflect their preferences, values, and comfort levels. Decision analysts take existing information about a medication's risks and benefits and calculate outcomes accordingly. We could not find any recent ones for HRT, but we did find two decision analyses conducted years ago, long before the Women's Health Initiative. One, done by Robin Gorsky in the department of health management and policy at the University of New Hampshire and her colleagues, concluded that the health benefits of postmenopausal estrogen exceeded the health risks. In their analysis, fifty-year-old women were assumed to take estrogen for twenty-five years, to age seventy-five. In a cohort of ten thousand women, those using estrogen would gain nearly four additional quality-adjusted years of life compared with women not using it.[47]

Another decision analysis was provided by Nananda Col and her colleagues, who concluded as early as 1997 that "hormone replacement therapy should increase life expectancy for nearly all postmenopausal women, with some gains exceeding 3 years, depending mainly on an individual's risk factors for CHD and breast cancer. For women with at least 1 risk factor for CHD, hormone therapy should extend life expectancy, even for women having first-degree relatives with breast cancer.... The benefit of hormone replacement therapy in reducing the likelihood of developing CHD appears to outweigh the risk of breast cancer for nearly all women in whom this treatment might be considered. Our analysis supports the broader use of hormone replacement therapy."[48] And her analysis was written before the onslaught of evidence showing that HRT does not increase the risk of breast cancer.

In sum, there is now a consensus that when taken at the start of menopause or before age sixty, HRT confers protection against coronary artery disease and heart attacks. What, however, is the "start of menopause"? Menopause is defined as the absence of periods for twelve months. But many women begin having menopause-related symptoms—such as insomnia, muscle pains, and heart palpitations—even when they are still menstruating, and HRT can benefit them too. Here is what we know:

- ERT or HRT may have beneficial effects on the heart for women who start taking hormones early in menopause because estrogen promotes healthy blood vessels and may help delay the formation of plaque.

- ERT or HRT probably has no protective effect on women who begin the use of hormones later, in their mid-sixties, although this conclusion is still being evaluated.
- ERT or HRT is potentially risky for women who begin taking it in their sixties, at least for the first year, especially if they have preexisting coronary artery disease.

At the 2017 American College of Cardiology's annual meeting, researchers at Cedars-Sinai Medical Center in Los Angeles reported their findings after analyzing the records of more than four thousand women who had been given a coronary calcium scan, an indirect measure of plaque buildup in the arteries, between 1998 and 2012. (We pause to note the influence of the Women's Health Initiative: more than 60 percent of these women were taking hormones in 1998, and only 23 percent in 2012.) After accounting for the women's ages, calcium scores, and cardiovascular risk factors, they found that women who had been taking HRT were 30 percent less likely to die than those not on hormone therapy; 36 percent were less likely to have a coronary calcium score above 399 (indicative of severe atherosclerosis and high heart attack risk); and 20 percent were more likely to have a coronary calcium score of 0 (the lowest possible score, indicating a low likelihood of heart attack).[49]

Three to four more years of healthy life with a much lower risk of heart disease? That's good enough evidence for us.

4

Breaking Bad

Avrum's mother-in-law, Charlotte, was standing alone outside on the granite entry to Av's office building. Without warning, her left hip gave way and she fell to the ground. She did not lose consciousness, nor did she feel much pain, but she was unable to get up. Charlotte was seventy-eight years old at the time and was found to have a fracture in the neck of her femur. She had no prior history of a hip injury, and it seemed that her femur had simply tired of supporting her weight. She was a healthy woman and no one, including Av, had predicted a vulnerability to fracture. On the contrary, she had dutifully taken vitamins and calcium for years and had been a champion handball player in her early life.

Osteoporosis, which means "porous bone," describes the cavities that develop in aging bones as they slowly degenerate. Bones that have been thinned out by these cavities are less able to support a person's weight, and if the bones become too thin and brittle, they can easily fracture—indeed, sometimes the simple act of bending over or even coughing will do it. Increasing bone fragility is a normal part of aging, just like cataracts, gray hair, and taking longer to recall the name of that guy you'll never forget. But osteoporosis is a different magnitude of bone loss—it's like the difference between the normal slowdown in retrieving that name and dementia.

The development of osteoporosis in later years affects men and women of all ethnicities, but the risks are higher among white and Asian women, women who are very thin, and women who enter menopause early. Women over the age of fifty have four times the rate of osteoporosis that men do, and their fractures occur five to ten years earlier than men's.[1] As people are living longer, hip fractures that result from osteoporosis are becoming more frequent, increasing at a rate of 1 to 3 percent per year in most areas of the world.[2] Of course, osteoporosis is not the only cause of hip fractures. A woman's risk doubles if her mother had a hip fracture before age eighty; other factors, such as poor eyesight and balance problems, increase the risk of falls in older people, which in turn increases the risk of fractures.[3]

Bones are living things. Like our hearts and muscles, they are not the same as they were last week or last year. Bones are in a constant state of equilibrium between the cells that build them up and those that break them down. Over a person's lifetime, that balance between growth and loss changes. Until the age of twenty-five, more bone is formed than lost. From twenty-five to thirty, women reach their peak bone mass, and that remains steady for the next decade. After women turn forty, bone formation slowly declines, and after they turn fifty, bone loss is greater than bone formation; osteoporosis is the cumulative result.

The areas in the skeletal system where thinning bones cause the most trouble are the spinal column and the hips. The spinal column is made up of twenty-four individual vertebrae extending from the neck to the low back and nine fused vertebrae in the sacrum and coccyx. Each individual vertebra is separated from its neighbor above and below by a spongy disk that helps absorb the thumps and assaults of everyday life and cushions the vertebral bone. Over the course of many years, however, the vertebrae develop tiny microfractures as a result of repeated small injuries and the usual stresses of life and are slowly compressed, thereby making us shorter as we get older. When the front-facing sides of the vertebrae at the neck or upper spine wear down faster than the back sides, the vertebrae tilt forward, creating the ill-named dowager's hump at the base of the neck and upper back—a sign of advanced osteoporosis. Exercises can correct bad posture (frequently caused by the forward slumping that so many people develop from hours at the computer), but they cannot fix the anatomy of degenerated bone.

A far more serious problem than fractures of the vertebrae are hip fractures that result from a gradual weakening of the largest bones in the body, the femurs, especially the necks of the femurs, which have the daunting task of supporting the weight of the upper half of the body. Hip fractures can cause immense pain and lasting disability; many of us can tell sorrowful stories of a healthy beloved older relative who was doing fine until she had an unexpected fall, broke her hip or pelvis, and subsequently sank into mental and physical decline.

Even more worrying, hip fractures increase the risk of death among older people. The most common estimates are that about 20 to 25 percent of the patients who have hip fractures, especially if they are in their seventies or eighties, will die within a year, and many more will suffer serious impairments in functioning.[4] In a major study headed by Danish endocrinologists, nearly 170,000 patients with hip fractures—virtually every patient in Denmark who broke a hip between 1977 and 2001—were compared with a control group, matched by age and gender, and followed for as long as twenty years from the date of injury. The mortality rate was twice as high in fracture cases as in the control group, primarily during the first year but continuing for the next five years. Perhaps that higher risk of death occurs because an old person who falls and breaks a hip is suffering from other age-related diseases? No. Although the fracture patients were more likely to have other medical problems, those problems did not affect their higher risk of death; the major reason for this higher rate was complications from the fracture. After having a hip fracture, women lost an average of 3.75 years of life. Rather dramatically, the researchers calculated that if the women were fifty or younger at the time of the fractures, they would lose 27 percent of their expected remaining years; if they were over eighty, they would lose 38 percent of their expected remaining years.[5]

Two large-scale international studies echoed these mortality results. In France, researchers followed 7,512 postmenopausal women for an average of four years. The women who had a first hip fracture during that time were four times more likely to die than were those who did not have a fracture—and, again, this increase in mortality was most pronounced during the first six months following the fracture.[6] In Sweden, researchers followed 1,013 hip-fracture patients and 2,026 matched controls for, incredibly, twenty-two years. Twenty-one percent of the female patients died within a year of the hip fracture compared to 6 percent of the controls, and the risk of death was more than doubled for at least ten years following the hip fracture. It remained at least 50 percent higher for the duration of the twenty-two-year observation period.[7]

Understandably, then, the prevalence of hip fractures and their consequences for impaired functioning and well-being are a major public health concern. Although rates of hip fractures have declined slightly since 1995 (for unknown reasons), the absolute numbers have increased along with the aging population. Women fear dying of breast cancer, but current estimates suggest that that risk and the lifetime risk of dying of the complications of a hip fracture are about the same.[8]

Bone Density versus Bone Resilience: A Crucial Distinction

The structure of bone is similar to the structure of a tall building. The girders that support the building are comparable to the collagen fibers within bone that provide, in addition to structural support, elasticity or tensile strength, allowing the bone to undergo stress, to bend without breaking. This flexible internal framework of the bone is called the osteoid. Calcium is deposited in and on the osteoid, creating the outer shell of the bone, like the external face of the building. The calcium in that outer shell provides a strong shield for the softer osteoid and aids the load-bearing potential of the bone, but it does not aid the bone's ability to bend without breaking.[9] An increase in calcium and other minerals, therefore, increases the stiffness and supportive strength of the bone but decreases its flexibility. As a woman ages, the thick, elastic collagen fibers inside the bone become thinner and more brittle. The tensile strength of the bone, which is a measurement of the force required to bend the bone to the point where it snaps, is diminished, and bone fractures occur more easily.

The first physician to advocate estrogen treatment to prevent osteoporosis was Fuller Albright, in 1940.[10] Albright was an honored endocrinologist who specialized in bone metabolism; to this day, the American Society for Bone and Mineral Research gives the Fuller Albright Award in recognition of outstanding accomplishment in the field. In 1946, Albright carefully distinguished *osteoporosis,* a disease caused by a lack of resilience within the matrix of the bone, from *osteomalacia* (known as rickets in children), caused by the bones' deficiency of minerals. With osteomalacia, the bones lack the strength conferred by calcium during a person's first two decades of life and bend on exposure to stress. (The bowlegged stance of children who grow up in impoverished areas and lack both vitamin D and calcium is characteristic of this condition.) Albright found that of his forty-two patients under age sixty-five who had osteoporosis in the spine and the hip, forty were postmenopausal women and only two were men. Accordingly, he named the condition *postmenopausal osteoporosis* to distinguish it from what he considered normal bone loss due to aging. But over the decades, as women began living many years past menopause and into their eighties and nineties, the condition he observed in his under-sixty-five-year-old women began to afflict many millions more.

Over time, however, some physicians began to conflate osteoporosis and osteomalacia, and the subsequent blurring of the two conditions led to the widespread but incorrect belief that if women just took enough calcium and vitamin D, they could stave off osteoporosis. It's easy to see how this mistake made its way into the culture. Even the National Library of Medicine's website advises women to take calcium and vitamins to ward off the risk of osteoporotic bone fractures.

Although calcium is crucial for the development of strong bones in children and adolescents, once bones are formed, additional calcium neither prevents nor treats bone loss. Albright had cautioned that because postmenopausal osteoporosis was not caused by any process related to the metabolism of calcium or other minerals, high intakes of these minerals with or without vitamin D would have no benefit. His observation was correct then, and it still is. In 2017, a team of orthopedic surgeons, headed by Jia-Guo Zhao at Tianjin Hospital in Tianjin, China, published a major meta-analysis in *JAMA*—thirty-three randomized trials involving 51,145 people—that compared the incidence of fractures in people taking supplements versus those taking a placebo or getting no treatment. They found absolutely no association between calcium on its own, vitamin D on its own, or calcium plus vitamin D and the incidence of nonvertebral, vertebral, or total fractures.[11]

The reason that calcium supplements do not reduce the risk of hip fractures is that they do not affect the interior architecture of the bone. According to randomized controlled studies and studies that follow cohorts of older people over time,[12] calcium supplements affect *density* but not *resilience*—the ability of bones to bend without breaking—and, as we said, it's resilience that matters here. That is the reason for the WHI's finding that calcium and vitamin D supplements resulted in a small improvement in hip-bone density. But because density does not equate with resilience, the supplements did not significantly reduce the incidence of hip fracture.[13]

Both estrogen and progesterone stimulate bone formation and inhibit bone loss, and, to date, no therapy studied has been better than ERT or HRT in preventing osteoporosis and fractures in the spine and hips. From the 1970s through the 1990s, estrogen was the cornerstone of the prevention and treatment of osteoporosis, whether on its own or in combination with progesterone.[14] A consensus development conference is a meeting of experts convened to assess the best medical approach to a particular problem. Two such conferences, one held at the NIH and one sponsored by the European Foundation for Osteoporosis and Bone Disease, reported that estrogen slowed or even stopped bone loss and was the only well-established treatment that reduced the frequency of osteoporotic fractures in postmenopausal women.[15] Studies at the Fred Hutchinson Cancer Research Center in Seattle and the long-running Framingham study found that postmenopausal women taking estrogen had a 35 to 50 percent reduction in the likelihood of having a fracture.[16] In the 1990s, three major studies in Sweden of many thousands of women likewise found that among those who were taking estrogen (ERT or HRT), the risk of having a first hip fracture was significantly reduced.[17]

The WHI investigators themselves acknowledged this benefit of estrogen. As early as 2002, they reported finding a 33 percent reduction in hip fractures among women on ERT or HRT. This finding was confirmed a decade later: 896 women (11.1 percent) in the placebo group had had fractures compared to 783 women (8.6 percent) in the estrogen-plus-progestin group.[18]

However, for estrogen to reduce the risk of fractures that occur ten to thirty years after menopause, postmenopausal women must be on HRT for at least ten years — and possibly for the rest of their lives. In a large clinical review of the evidence in 2005, Nananda Col and her colleagues noted that because 86 percent of hip fractures occur among women over the age of sixty-five, women who take hormones only in their fifties, typically to alleviate menopausal symptoms, would not derive much benefit in terms of protecting their bones decades later. A few years of taking hormones, they said, would have little effect on fracture risk by the time a woman approaches the age at which that risk peaks.[19] They were right; the protective effect of hormone therapy on the bones vanishes when it is stopped, and bone loss resumes at an accelerated rate.[20] When women go off estrogen, the risk of hip fractures rapidly increases, and within six years it is where it would have been had they never taken hormones at all.

In a review of eleven studies of estrogen and hip fracture published since 1990, epidemiologist Deborah Grady and her colleagues at the University of California, San Francisco, found that all but one reported a reduction in the risk of hip fractures among women taking estrogen compared with nonusers. Again, the longer the women had been taking estrogen — ten years or more — the lower their risk of hip fractures.[21] And, again, that beneficial effect, even among women who had been taking estrogen for a decade, declined rapidly after they stopped. Women ages sixty-five to seventy-four who had taken estrogen in the past had a 63 percent reduction in the risk of hip fracture, but if they stopped taking hormones, by the time they were seventy-five, they had only an 18 percent reduction in risk. A year after this study came out, Grady and her colleague Bruce Ettinger, an osteoporosis specialist and endocrinologist, concluded: "To provide maximal protection, estrogen treatment may have to be started at the time of the menopause and never stopped."[22]

The primary reason that hormones were unseated as the method of choice for preventing or delaying osteoporosis was, no surprise, the WHI-inspired fear that HRT caused breast cancer. Even today, the Mayo Clinic's website states that "the reduction of estrogen levels in women around the time of menopause is one of the strongest risk factors for developing osteoporosis.... Estrogen, especially when started soon after menopause, can help maintain bone density." Then, regrettably, it adds: "However, estrogen therapy can increase the risk of blood clots, endometrial cancer, breast cancer and possibly heart disease."[23] As we have seen, that caution is largely unwarranted. Nevertheless, aren't there alternatives to hormones that prevent severe bone loss in old age and reduce the likelihood of hip fractures and their attendant risks?

WHAT ARE THE ALTERNATIVES?

Many health activists and historians of medicine believe that osteoporosis is not as serious a concern as it has been made out to be. After all, the vast majority of women, even in their eighties, will not suffer hip fractures, although they likely will have age-related microfractures in the spine. But losing a few inches in height hardly warrants a woman taking hormones her whole postmenopausal life, they argue. In *Aging Bones: A Short History of Osteoporosis,* medical historian Gerald N. Grob told the story of how, in his view, the "normal aging of bones was transformed into a medical diagnosis that eventually included every aged person."[24] This transformation, he maintained, occurred "through a coalition of cultural, medical and pharmaceutical forces that moved osteoporosis from the margins of health research in the earlier part of the twentieth century to the centre of a national and well-funded American agenda by the twenty-first century, that urged all women over 65 (and men over 70) to be screened for bone mineral density (BMD)." Grob showed how during the 1950s and 1960s, as more and more people were living to the age of sixty-five and beyond, older people "emerged as a self-conscious group with distinct interests," one of which was a vehement rejection of viewing old age solely as a gloomy time of infirmity and disability. Nonetheless, older people found themselves facing new health concerns created by additional years of life. "Preventing age-related decline," wrote Grob, "became a focus for researchers and clinicians alike."

Grob had no quarrel with efforts to help old people live healthier lives; his concern was society's labeling the normal changes that occur with age, including menopause and bone loss, as diagnosable "diseases." Osteoporosis and its treatment, Grob argued, were "shaped by illusions about the conquest of disease and aging. These illusions, in turn, are instrumental in shaping our health care system. While bone density tests and osteoporosis treatments are now routinely prescribed, aggressive pharmaceutical intervention has produced results that are inconclusive at best."

We fully agree with Grob in his assessment of the cultural manufacture of new diseases that allegedly warrant drugs that Big Pharma just coincidentally happens to have developed. We too lament the American pursuit of youth and the illusions of conquering age. But the search for treatments to help the millions who are at risk of suffering or premature death, precisely because they are living longer than would once have been dreamed possible, is another matter entirely. Alzheimer's disease and other forms of dementia also afflict people living into old age; should we not do all we can to understand the causes of these disorders and thereby prevent or treat them?

For their part, many women are uncomfortable with the idea of taking any medication for their entire lives after menopause. Even Ettinger and Grady, who found that improvement in bone resilience conferred by estrogen was likely to reduce the risk of fracture by about two-thirds, worried that "having to take estrogen for the rest of one's life reduces the appeal of this preventive strategy." Some writers suggest that only women at very high risk of bone fractures (as we noted, that group includes white women, Asian women, very thin women, women who entered menopause early, and women whose mothers had hip fractures) should consider HRT. Everyone else should look first to alternatives: Exercise. Lose weight. Take fluoride. Take calcium. Take medication designed to prevent osteoporosis, namely bisphosphonates.[25] If only it were that easy.

Exercise, the most popular recommended alternative to hormones for bone strength, is a fine activity for many health reasons; weight training in particular is of undeniable benefit to women as they age. Some investigators have suggested that peak bone strength can be achieved by a combination of exercise and calcium during a woman's premenopausal years, while she has adequate levels of circulating estrogen, and that an elevated peak bone strength might stave off or delay future osteoporosis. While exercise may improve bone strength and resistance to fracture in *premenopausal* women, however, it does not improve bone strength or resistance to fracture among *postmenopausal* women who are not on HRT.[26]

Because fluoride protects the outer shell of our teeth, some investigators have tried it as a treatment for women with osteoporosis, administering it in large doses to prevent further deterioration of bones. Fluoride does generate dramatic increases in bone density but it does not improve bone tensile strength, probably because it makes the bones less flexible. The risk of nonvertebral fractures actually increases with the use of fluoride treatments.[27] (But don't stop using your fluoride toothpaste.)

Well, then, what alternatives might increase bone flexibility? Bone density can be measured, but the more relevant bone fragility—the bones' response to tensile stress—cannot. The best way to test the tensile strength of bone would be to clamp the bone in a vise and determine how much bending the bone could tolerate before it breaks. Clearly, this is not a practical method! Physicians therefore use a bone mineral density (BMD) test as a substitute for measuring the tensile strength of bone, but they often overlook the fact that this test is an inaccurate measure of fracture risk.[28] Today the most commonly used test is dual-energy X-ray absorptiometry (DXA), which uses X-rays to measure the amounts of calcium and other minerals in the bone. But it too is measuring bone density, not bone resilience.

BMD tests were supported by the pharmaceutical industry, and

Gerry Grob, along with other bioethicists, medical historians, and consumer advocates, warned that once the tests were in widespread use, they would open the door for new medications for osteoporosis.[29] Before a company can sell a drug, after all, it must have a condition or disease that the medication treats. Therefore, it must have a way of identifying that disease. And if a company can cast a wide net in its definition of that disease, it'll have an even larger market of people to take its new drug. But where along the continuum of bone loss—which, after all, happens to everyone—does it become a disease? How little is too much?

The ensuing commercial campaign to simplify the decision to prescribe medication began with an arbitrary answer: on the continuum of bone loss, a person whose bone mineral density test score is 2.5 standard deviations below that of a healthy thirty-year-old will meet the (artificial) diagnosis of osteoporosis. (A standard deviation is a statistical measure that describes the distance, or deviation, from the norm.) In the early 1990s, this numerical criterion was endorsed by the World Health Organization, and with that official imprimatur, researchers and clinicians had a tangible number to hold on to.[30] That –2.5 diagnostic threshold, wrote Bruce Ettinger and his colleagues, was simply a benchmark for estimating the prevalence of osteoporosis across various countries. "It was not intended," they wrote, "to be the sole clinical criterion for determining drug treatment. Intervention thresholds differ from diagnostic thresholds."[31]

But wait—if –2.5 is bad, isn't –2.0 or –1.5 pre-bad? What if your score is less than that normal thirty-year-old's but not officially osteoporotic? That can't be good for you, can it? Accordingly, the term *osteopenia* emerged, defined as a BMD test result between

–1.0 and –2.5 standard deviations below that of a healthy thirty-year-old. Osteopenia was assumed to be an inevitable precursor of osteoporosis, just as a puppy is a pre-dog. The World Health Organization emphasized that this diagnostic category was not meant to be used in clinical practice, because *osteopenia* has no clinical significance and does not even predict the risk for osteoporotic fracture. Canadian physicians and health-policy specialists Angela Cheung and Allan Detsky reported that a history of falls is a stronger predictor of fractures than bone mineral density results, which do not correlate well with the risk of hip fracture.[32] The term *osteopenia* has "no medical meaning," Steven Cummings, an epidemiologist who has conducted numerous large-scale studies, told a reporter. "I've seen patients who come in scared that they will become disabled soon because they have this 'disease' called osteopenia, when in fact they are normal for their age."[33] Nortin M. Hadler, professor of medicine and microbiology/immunology at the University of North Carolina at Chapel Hill and author of several books on medical overtreatment, was even more forthright. "Osteopenia is an example of a New Age social construction," he said, adding that it was invented and sustained by marketers, drug companies, and others with vested interests.[34]

Too late for the warnings; there's too much money at stake. Gynecologists began buying expensive DXA machines to use on their patients; Carol's doctor told her she had osteopenia but then had the grace to laugh and say, "Although that doesn't mean anything." Prescriptions for bisphosphonates, seen as an alternative to HRT to ward off bone loss, skyrocketed, used to treat both the meaningless osteopenia and the true condition of osteoporosis. Ever since the Women's Health Initiative, the preventive treatment of osteoporosis has been dominated by nonhormonal bisphospho-nates such as Fosamax, Aredia, Actonel, Zometa, Reclast, and Boniva.[35] These come in oral and intravenous forms and can be taken daily, weekly, monthly, or even annually. Bisphosphonates do nothing for the nonexistent condition of osteopenia, but they can avert osteoporosis in women at high risk and also stabilize bone loss in women who already have it. Once osteoporosis has devel-oped, however, it is highly unlikely that the drugs can reverse the condition.

The side effects of the bisphosphonates can be unpleasant, and some are far worse than those for hormones. The most common are abdominal discomfort, muscle or joint pain, fever and flulike symp-toms, and insomnia; two very rare but devastating side effects are kidney damage and osteonecrosis of the jaw, a disease presumed to be caused by a diminished flow of blood to the bone in that area. No wonder that among patients with osteoporosis, including those who have had fractures, 70 percent stop the medication within a year.[36]

Worse, paradoxically, when the bisphosphonates are taken for long periods, they have been associated with an *increased* risk of atypical hip fractures. Unlike hip fractures caused by osteoporosis, which usually occur at the angled upper extension (the neck) of the femur, atypical femoral fractures generally develop below the femo-ral neck in the upper part of the shaft. There is growing evidence that taking bisphosphonates over the long term may impair the bones' ability to repair microcracks, thereby leading to increased skeletal fragility.[37] In 2017, the Women's Health Initiative con-cluded that in older women at high risk of fracture, taking bio-phosphates for ten to thirteen years was associated with a higher risk of clinical fracture than two years of use.[38]

All of this evidence led Robert Langer, a principal WHI investigator (whose criticism of its initial reports we described in chapter 1), to argue that estrogen was a better preventive: "Unlike bisphosphonates, which have been associated with excessive bone mineralization, estrogen facilitates normal bone architecture. There is no question that estrogen is an effective and metabolically appropriate preventive strategy for osteoporotic fractures, and that osteoporosis is a chronic disease with tremendous impact in postmenopausal women."[39]

The pharmaceutical industry is not sitting around quietly resting on its bisphosphonates, you can be sure. Many drug companies have entered the race for other ways to prevent or treat osteoporosis. Consider these alternatives to bisphosphonates:

Raloxifene (Evista), a SERM (selective estrogen-receptor modulator), is prescribed for some postmenopausal, estrogen-receptor-positive breast cancer survivors to decrease the risk of breast cancer recurrence. Raloxifene has been used to treat osteoporosis for many years, but researchers have known for two decades that although it does decrease the risk of vertebral fractures, it does not reduce the risk of hip fractures.[40] About a fourth of the women who take it report hot flashes, and 10 to 20 percent report flulike symptoms, sinusitis, joint pains, and muscle spasms.

Calcitonin, a hormone produced in the thyroid gland, helps regulate the blood's calcium and phosphate levels. It is generally administered by nasal spray or injection. It may help reduce bone loss, but there is no substantive evidence that it reduces the risk of fractures.[41]

Teriparatide (Forteo), a form of parathyroid hormone generated from recombinant DNA, has not been extensively studied, but early reports suggest it stimulates bone growth and reduces the risk of hip fractures in patients who have already developed osteoporosis.[42] However, its protective effects wane after two years of continued treatment. Abaloparatide, a chemical cousin of Forteo, has been shown to reduce both vertebral and hip fractures, but its effectiveness over time has not yet been studied.[43]

Denosumab (marketed as Prolia or Xgeva), approved for the treatment of osteoporosis and to decrease fractures caused by metastases of cancer to the bone, has a similar rate of success as the bisphosphonates in reducing the risk of vertebral and hip fractures and must be taken indefinitely. But few patients are willing to do that. Nearly half of the women who take this drug report side effects of fatigue and weakness; about 20 percent report shortness of breath, coughing, and muscle and joint pain. A dangerous drop in calcium levels has been reported in 4 percent of cancer patients treated with denosumab.[44]

Of all these efforts to develop the best drug, the story of romosozumab is perhaps the most instructive. Romosozumab, developed by Celltech and marketed by Amgen, binds to and inhibits sclerostin, a protein that leads to bone resorption (loss). There was great excitement in 2017 when a study of the drug that included nearly 4,100 postmenopausal women with osteoporosis and clinically determined evidence of a fragility fracture was published in the *New England Journal of Medicine*. The accompanying editorial was titled "Romosozumab—Promising or Practice Changing?" The women were randomly assigned to receive the newer drug or Fosamax for twelve months, followed by another year of Fosamax for everyone. The researchers then looked to see how many women had developed new fractures at twenty-four months. The results sure seemed "practice changing." After two years, the romosozumab-to-Fosamax group had nearly half the risk of developing new vertebral fractures (6.2 percent) than the Fosamax-only group (11.9 percent), and a lower risk of hip fractures as well.[45]

The research was funded by Amgen. In that same year, the FDA rejected the drugmaker's application for approval because the drug also caused an increased risk of "serious adverse cardiovascular events." As one news report noted:

> Safety concerns could limit the label of romosozumab and in doing so dent its blockbuster ambitions. "Ultimately based on a label that fits the right risk/benefit population and based on conversations with Amgen, we still think the drug could be a $500M+ franchise," Jefferies analyst Michael Yee wrote in a note to investors. The situation makes romosozumab part of an emerging clutch of Amgen drugs that have run into trouble — or look likely to do so — when trying to transition from promising clinical prospects to commercial successes.[46]

Did you get that "blockbuster ambitions" part? The drug company is regrouping and appealing the FDA decision.

THE TAKE-HOME

We are mindful of the irony that, while we are busy criticizing Big Pharma for hurrying new drugs to market, exaggerating their benefits, and minimizing their risks, we are advocating the use of HRT and ERT, both of which are manufactured by Big Pharma companies. We are not happy that Wyeth, which has held the patent on Premarin for sixty years, has fought in court to prevent generic formulations from being marketed. Because Wyeth controls this drug, which is the most widely prescribed estrogen, it has been able to increase its price. We deplore this action, by Wyeth or any other drug company. But reprehensible marketing practices do not necessarily negate a drug's benefits, and Premarin's safety and efficacy record stretches back for decades.

As an oncologist and hematologist who has been in medical practice for fifty years, Avrum knows full well that no physician can read and evaluate every article that appears in the medical literature and that some research will be inconsistent with the conclusions that he or she comes to. In the case of HRT's benefits for bone health, his conclusions are the result of a lifetime of assessing findings from published research, his accumulated clinical experience, his debates with respected colleagues, and the constant input from his peers and his patients. Given present knowledge, he feels that these conclusions are warranted:

- Osteoporosis and subsequent bone fracture with resulting disability and death are growing problems for the expanding population of women living into their seventies, eighties, and nineties.
- Currently, ERT or HRT is the most effective intervention with the fewest unpleasant or dire side effects for preventing or diminishing the development of osteoporosis. It has been repeatedly shown to reduce the risk of the condition's most incapacitating complication, hip fracture, by 30 to 50 per-

cent. In absolute numbers, this reduction is highly meaningful.

- Exercise may improve bone strength and resistance to fracture in premenopausal women, but it does not improve bone strength or resistance to fracture among postmenopausal women who are not on HRT.
- Calcium supplements, which millions of women take in hopes of fending off loss of bone density, are ineffective in preventing postmenopausal osteoporosis or fractures because they do not affect bone *resilience.*
- The most frequently prescribed nonhormonal osteoporosis medications, the bisphosphonates, are associated with gastrointestinal discomfort, fatigue, and insomnia; with an increased risk of atypical femoral fractures if taken for a long time; and with the rare but debilitating development of kidney problems or osteonecrosis of the jaw.

The prevention of osteoporosis may not be the leading and best reason for women to take HRT; Gerry Grob and other critics of medicalization are right, after all, that the vast majority of women will not develop this condition nor die of it. But the research persuades us that women who are at high risk of osteoporosis should continue taking hormones indefinitely once they are past menopause. And for those who decide to take HRT for the many other benefits it confers, having stronger and more resilient bones certainly seems to be one hell of a welcome side effect.

5

Losing and Using Our Minds

I t was an ominous headline, which was why it was so effective. There it was, in huge type on the front page of the Sunday Review section of the November 19, 2017, *New York Times:* "Is Alzheimer's Coming for You?" Followed by the slug: "Simple blood tests may soon be able to deliver alarming news about your cognitive health." Oh, goody.

The article sure grabbed our attention. It reported that anywhere from one-fourth to one-half of the population will show signs of Alzheimer's disease by age eighty-five, a risk that is even higher among people carrying one or two copies of the gene variant APOE4 (apolipoprotein E4). The article raised the possibility of a future blood test that would be easier and less expensive than gene sequencing, a test that could identify pre-Alzheimer's in forty- to fifty-year-old people who have no obvious symptoms. Pagan Kennedy, the reporter, interviewed research scientists who were studying Alzheimer's causes as well as people who knew they had the gene variant and had joined support groups, seeking diet and life-style interventions in hopes of preventing or at least slowing the progression of the disease. One neurologist, David Holtzman, had been studying the APOE gene for twenty-five years without look-ing to see if he had the APOE4 variant. When Kennedy asked him why he hadn't, he told her there was no point because there was no drug or lifestyle program guaranteed to protect the brain.

Alzheimer's disease is one of many conditions that fall under the umbrella term *dementia*. Right behind women's fear of breast cancer is the fear of "losing it": losing memory, clear thinking, words. (A fear that men share, of course.) Everyone becomes for-getful: "Where are those keys? Why did I come into the den—was I looking for something?" Cognitive slowdown is normal as we age; we *will* remember the name of that actor who played the rock star in *Almost Famous** or, hell, a movie we saw last week, but it will take us longer than we'd like. Mild cognitive slowdown is variously exasperating and amusing, but for people entering their sixties and seventies, the prospect of dementia is terrifying: "If I can't remem-ber now where I put my car keys, does that mean that one day I won't remember what car keys are for?" Many people fear so, but these are very different matters. A sign of dementia is memory loss that disrupts daily life: forgetting recently learned information and important dates, asking for the same information over and over, relying on family members for reminders of events the person could once easily handle. But merely forgetting names or appointments for a while and remembering them eventually are typical changes that occur with age.

---

* Billy Crudup.

In 1900, only 5 percent of all American women lived beyond their fiftieth birthday;[1] today their average life expectancy has reached eighty years. For women now age forty-five, the estimated lifetime risk for developing Alzheimer's dementia is one in five; it's one in ten for men. One reason for women's higher risk is their longer life span, since rates of Alzheimer's dementia increase dramatically with age; but even after controlling for their greater longevity, women are still more likely than men to develop the disease. Almost two-thirds of all people with Alzheimer's are women, and a woman in her sixties is twice as likely to develop Alzheimer's as she is to develop breast cancer.[2] Because the overall population continues to age, with more and more people living well past their eighties, the number of people who die from Alzheimer's disease every year has almost doubled even while deaths from other diseases—notably breast cancer, prostate cancer, stroke, and heart disease—are in decline. As a 2017 report from the Alzheimer's Association noted, someone in the United States develops Alzheimer's disease every sixty-six seconds, and by 2050, barring scientific discoveries, it will be one new case every thirty-three seconds.[3]

Because Alzheimer's patients typically survive from four to ten years after the onset of the illness, the cost of their care to families and society is immense, financially as well as emotionally. With about five and a half million Americans living with Alzheimer's, the total cost for their health care, including long-term care and hospice services, has surpassed the quarter-trillion mark: $259 billion.[4] (For comparison, that is about $100 billion more than the cost of care for people with all cancers combined.)

Given the suffering that Alzheimer's disease causes, the misery it inflicts on families, and the financial burden it imposes, it's no wonder that attempts to prevent it, control it, and treat it are a high priority. Scientists are investigating all kinds of possible causes, including genetics, exposure to environmental toxins and pollution, cardiovascular problems, and chronic inflammation. And yet almost nothing is known for sure. Because the only way to accurately diagnose it is by microscopic assessment of the brain after death, the diagnosis of the disease in living persons is not definitive. Alzheimer's might prove to be a family of illnesses rather than one.

To date, the *Times'* interviewee David Holtzman is right that no treatment is truly effective in preventing the development of dementia. The FDA has approved some drugs to ease the symptoms of Alzheimer's dementia: donepezil (Aricept), mirtazapine (Remeron), tacrine (Cognex, which was discontinued in the United States because of its link with acute liver damage), galantamine (Reminyl or Razadyne), rivastigmine (Exelon), memantine (Ebixa or Namenda), and Namzaric, which combines donepezil with memantine. None of them slows or stops the progression of Alzheimer's disease.[5] In 2018, *JAMA* published the unhappy results of three international randomized clinical trials of yet another drug, idalopirdine; all found the drug had no benefit at all.[6]

And yet there is evidence that a powerful preventive, at least for women, is right under our noses: estrogen. Decades of research have demonstrated the role of estrogen in helping to preserve the cognitive ability of postmenopausal women and in decreasing the risk of Alzheimer's.[7] And then, in 2003, a team of WHI investigators published the results of the WHI Memory Study (WHIMS) and reported that estrogen plus progestin nearly doubled the relative risk for dementia in women sixty-five and older — further support, they said, for their warning that the risks of HRT outweighed any possible benefits.[8] That's frightening news indeed. Doubled the risk? Well, the investigators admitted, "the absolute risk is relatively small." The risk increased from 1 percent (21 out of 2,303) of the women on placebo to 1.8 percent (40 out of 2,229) of the women on HRT.

That was enough. In one fell swoop, all of the accumulated knowledge disputing that conclusion was rejected in favor of a small statistical finding of questionable significance, and millions of women were denied the potential benefit of HRT in warding off the cognitive decline that so often accompanies aging.

Still, nearly double is nearly double, so let's look closely at the basis of the WHI's claim. At the outset, the researchers had an admirable goal: They would select 8,300 women, all over age sixty-five, from the original, much larger WHI sample to be part of their memory study. (Thus, these women were not representative of the vast majority of women in the general population; most women who decide to take hormones usually start them when they enter menopause.) They would follow these women for five years to see who developed cognitive impairments and whether hormones increased their risk. The large size of the group—more than eight thousand—would allow them to draw statistically reliable conclusions.

However, this ambition was thwarted, because when the WHI ended the HRT part of the trial early, with those stop-the-presses claims of having found an increased risk of breast cancer, they had just 4,532 women enrolled. Of that number, only 61 women had developed dementia over four years. Undeterred by the few cases that might throw their calculations into question, the researchers justified the low number as being "in keeping with both the age of the cohort and the expectation that healthier, cognitively and behaviorally competent women were more likely to have enrolled in this complex and rigorously conducted clinical trial."[9] This is hardly a satisfying explanation for many reasons, starting with the fact that the great majority of the women in their sample were *not* healthier. (You may recall that 70 percent were overweight or obese, half were smokers, and many had hypertension.) Whatever the reason for the low number of women who developed dementia during the study, it means that any difference between the HRT group and the placebo group — that 1 percent versus 1.8 percent — could be statistically significant while at the same time being neither compelling nor clinically relevant.

The investigators claimed to have identified an elephant that on closer inspection turned out to be a mouse. Here is one of our favorite lines: "In the WHIMS," the authors began, and then they paused midsentence to interject a self-congratulatory pat on the back — "the first double-blind, placebo-controlled, long-term multicenter study of [ERT and HRT] in postmenopausal women" — *both* ERT and HRT "were associated with an increased incidence of dementia compared with placebo." That sounds bad, but the sentence continued: "although the association did not reach statistical significance in the smaller, but longer, estrogen-alone trial."[10] Talking out of both sides of their mouths in a single sentence, they told us there was an "increased incidence," but never mind, it was not significant for the estrogen users. What about women taking combined estrogen and progestin? Now they trumpeted that nearly doubled relative risk while acknowledging that the absolute risk was very low. But then they told us the increased risk appeared during the first year that women were taking HRT, suggesting that many of these participants already had cognitive decline at the start of the study. That means the investigators were fully aware that their tested population was perhaps not quite as healthy as they had boasted.

Trying to sort out the WHI's conclusions about estrogen and cognitive function is like playing a game of whack-a-mole: bop one of their overblown risks on the head, and another pops up somewhere else. Sometimes the investigators talked about "dementia," sometimes "mild cognitive impairment," and sometimes, grandly, "global cognitive function." Sometimes they twisted their data into contortions to eke out a finding. In 2004, when the investigators reported that women taking estrogen alone did not have an increased risk of dementia, they combined them with women taking estrogen and progestin—that is, they pooled the data from both groups— and in this way, they could report a slight increased risk of dementia for both.[11] How can that be so if the women on estrogen alone didn't have a greater risk?

As for that slightly increased risk of dementia for women on HRT: Most damning for the WHI's assertion, in that first 2003 report, there was no increased incidence of mild cognitive impairment between the HRT and placebo groups. This presented a problem: Given that "mild cognitive impairment" precedes the emergence of full-blown dementia, how could HRT cause the more serious disease but not its less serious precursor? If HRT were really harmful to the brain, surely mild cognitive problems would emerge first—the warning warble of a canary in a mental mine.

The following year, 2004, the investigators must have heard that warble. This time they decided to look at the women's "global cognitive function." ERT and HRT, they reported, were indeed associated with cognitive impairments, *but only among women who were already cognitively impaired at the outset.* When women who had mild cognitive impairment at the start of the study were excluded from analysis, the results were no longer statistically significant.[12] "No other factors appear to markedly influence the treatment effects of [HRT] or pooled hormone therapy," they wrote. "Among women whose scores exceeded 95 [normal cognitive ability], the mean decrement was small and not statistically different from zero."[13]

Translation: The cognitively healthy women on HRT did not become cognitively impaired!

Within a year, many of the WHI's critics had mobilized. Leon Speroff, an obstetrician-gynecologist whom we quoted in chapter 3, noted that "in the canceled estrogen-progestin arm of the WHI, the only increase in dementia was in the group of women who were 75 years and older when they started treatment."[14] Somehow that finding got lost in the WHI's press releases about women's dementia risks on HRT. Neuroscientists at the University of North Texas James Simpkins and Meharvan Singh, along with a team of neurobiologists, endocrinologists, and clinical scientists who specialized in estrogen research (including Roberta Brinton, Pauline Maki, and Barbara Sherwin), wrote a position paper critical of the WHI's claims. They observed that the results flew in the face of hundreds of studies conducted over a decade, many cited by the WHI investigators themselves, suggesting that estrogen could protect brain cells from damage and improve cognition in people and animals. The finding of the WHI memory study, they said, had been greatly exaggerated; the small increase in dementia risk could not be extended to all forms of HRT or even to the women most likely to start HRT.[15]

Once again, it seems that the WHI investigators were doing their best to interpret their elusive findings in the most negative way, and they were doing so by manipulating the numbers, redefining the outcomes (mild impairment to dementia to "global cognitive function"), and claiming that HRT caused cognitive impairments for all women rather than, specifically, for the very old and those who already had cognitive deficits. This was especially curious because they began their first paper with a litany of studies demonstrating estrogen's protective effects on the brain, including its ability to reduce the loss of neurons, improve cerebral blood flow, and modulate expression of the APOE gene.[16] Eventually, the WHI investigators conceded that their study was not designed to determine whether women who began taking estrogen at the time of menopause would have a lower risk of the onset of cognitive decline or Alzheimer's disease a decade or two later.[17] And they even agreed that "there may be a critical period during which hormone therapy must be initiated to protect cognitive functioning."[18] As we will see, there most certainly is.

Unfortunately, the worry that HRT increases the risk of dementia has survived among numerous physicians, even those who now recognize the limitations of many of the WHI's other scare findings. "My doctor won't prescribe HRT for me," one of Av's former patients, whom we will call Sarah, wrote to him. "He now agrees that it doesn't cause breast cancer, but he told me that the WHI found that it increases the risk of dementia, and he wants to protect me from that." Protect her? Didn't this physician speak to her? If he had, he might have learned that Sarah had been on hormones for many years and that she was, at age seventy-eight, still running her own demanding business.

Was estrogen a contributor to Sarah's healthy mental functioning, or does Sarah just have good genes, good workouts, and good habits? Scientists have three ways of investigating that question: they examine the anatomical and neurological changes in the brain that occur with impaired cognition and that estrogen might influence; they do research on animals; and they conduct human studies that examine the effects of estrogen on women's thinking and abilities in real life.

LESSONS FROM LABS

During the final third of the twentieth century, medical students were taught that human beings were born with a finite number of brain neurons (nerve cells), that the huge number of glial cells that surrounded them had no function other than to support the neurons in some vague way, that neurons did not divide or regenerate, and that everyone irreplaceably lost countless numbers of them every day. We now know that all of these claims are wrong. Brain neurons are capable of dividing and regenerating, and brain function depends crucially not only on neurons but also on the glial cells. *Glia* is from the Greek word for "glue," but these cells do more than glue neurons together. They provide the neurons with nutrients, insulate them, help them grow, protect the brain from toxic agents, and remove cellular debris when neurons die. They have even been found to evolve into neurons.[19] Without glia, neurons could not function effectively. Over time, glia help determine which neural connections get stronger or weaker, suggesting that they play a vital role in learning and memory.*

One of the most astonishing advances in brain science has been the discovery of the human brain's *neuroplasticity,* the fact that neurons can form new connections throughout a person's life, sometimes compensating for injury or disease. Laboratory studies have suggested that estrogen can enhance neuroplasticity by modifying the structure of nerve cells in the brain and altering the way they communicate with one another. The real-life applications of this research remain uncertain, but we want to describe here some of the abundant evidence that estrogen, administered when menopause begins, may prevent, or at least delay, the onset of dementia, including dementia resulting from Alzheimer's disease. As we noted in chapter 2, estrogen levels drop dramatically in women after menopause, to levels that are only about 1 percent of those in premenopausal women.[20] If estrogen is playing a role in protecting the brain's neurons and glia, and if that drop in estrogen is one of the major contributors to women's higher rate of Alzheimer's, it behooves us to pay attention.

Consider the kinds of anatomical aberrations that are found in the brains of patients with Alzheimer's disease. Although researchers still disagree about whether these aberrations directly cause Alzheimer's, they have identified brain pathology in specific areas involved in memory: the prefrontal cortex (active during short-term memory, and the part of the brain involved in planning and

---

* Scientists also used to think that the human brain contained about a hundred billion neurons and ten times as many glia. But recent advances have allowed researchers to count individual cells, and they put the numbers much lower; an adult brain contains around 171 billion cells, about evenly divided between neurons and glia.

higher mental functions), the hippocampus and related areas responsible for learning and retrieving stored information, and the amygdala (involved in forming, retrieving, and consolidating emotional memories). A person can have profound abnormalities in these areas and still be able to walk, talk, and taste without remembering the name of the person sitting across the dinner table. These pathological findings include the following:

- The death of nerve cells and a decreased density of those cells;
- Thinning and atrophy of the dendrites and axons, which extend outward from the body of a nerve cell like the arms of an octopus, conveying signals that allow nerve cells to communicate with one another;
- A decreased number of synapses (the connections between neurons);
- Neurofibrillary tangles, a primary marker of Alzheimer's; these are clusters of twisted fibers inside the neurons that consist primarily of a protein called tau, which is involved in transporting nutrients from one part of the neuron to another;
- Amyloid plaques, another Alzheimer's marker (clusters of disintegrated protein fragments that build up between nerve cells);
- Decreased stores within the neuron of acetylcholine, a chemical that allows messages to leap from one neuron to the next in regions of the memory centers of the brain, especially the hippocampus, and in other regions that affect memory and emotion. Patients with Alzheimer's disease have up to a 90 percent reduction in the level of this neurotransmitter;
- Dysfunctions of the glial cells.

Estrogen affects all of these aspects of brain anatomy, both directly and indirectly. It stimulates the growth of neurons and synapses, and it increases plasticity, the brain's remarkable ability to adapt and change.[21]

It turns out that estrogen receptors are located throughout the brain, especially in the hippocampus and other areas involved in learning and memory.[22] Neuroscientists such as Elizabeth Gould, who is now at the Princeton Neuroscience Institute, have found that estrogen affects the brain mechanisms involved in memory, aging, and degenerative diseases in various ways.[23] In one early study, for example, Gould and her colleagues found that removing the ovaries of adult female rats—which caused levels of circulating estrogen to plummet—resulted in a profound decrease in the number of dendrites on neurons in the rats' hippocampi. When they gave the rats estrogen, with or without progesterone, after removing the ovaries, this decrease did not occur.[24] Similarly, others have found that when female rats are given estrogen, the number of synapses within the hippocampus increases, they learn to run through mazes more quickly (and remember where the food is), and their neurons, especially those involved in memory, are more likely to survive during normal aging or exposure to toxins. Treating female rats with estrogen prolongs their survival, improves their spatial-recognition memory, and decreases the amount of amyloid in neurons.[25]

Roberta Diaz Brinton, another leading neuroscientist in this field, runs a research lab at the University of Arizona, where she studies the aging female brain and, in particular, how to prevent or delay Alzheimer's. In studies comparing estrogen-treated cells to cells not exposed to estrogen, she found significantly greater growth of dendrites and axons among the estrogen-treated cells as well as enhanced connections among brain cells.[26]

Estrogen has even more benefits for the brain:

- Estrogen increases the levels of an enzyme needed to synthesize acetylcholine.[27]
- Estrogen stimulates the growth of nerve cells, regenerates axons, and decreases the nerve-cell death that happens in Alzheimer's.[28]
- Estrogen protects nerve cells by preventing a dangerous accumulation of calcium within the cells.[29]
- Estrogen makes brain cells more responsive and sensitive to the effects of nerve growth factor (NGF), a protein responsible for the development of new neurons and the health of mature ones.[30] NGF increases the proliferation and density of nerve cells and stimulates the development of dendrites and axons. (NGF was discovered in the 1950s by the pioneering Italian neurobiologist Rita Levi-Montalcini, who, with her colleague Stanley Cohen, won a Nobel Prize for this work.)
- Estrogen reduces the production of beta amyloid, the substance that accumulates in amyloid plaques. It also protects brain cells against damage by beta amyloid.[31]
- Estrogen prevents the buildup of the tau protein.[32]
- Estrogen enhances the action of glial cells.[33]
- Estrogen enhances the ability of neurons to survive toxic insults by,[34] for example, stimulating glial cells to regulate inflammatory responses after brain injury.
- Estrogen improves cerebral blood flow. In women who have extremely low estrogen levels because of illness or surgery,

their blood-flow patterns resemble those of patients with mild to moderate Alzheimer's. In one study, it was found that administering estrogen reversed these detrimental blood-flow changes and restored a normal pattern after only six weeks.[35]

- Estrogen promotes the uptake of glucose and its metabolism in the brain. When women begin going through menopause and estrogen declines, so do the glucose levels in their brains. Why does this matter? Although the brain takes up only 2 percent of a person's body weight, it uses some 20 percent of the body's glucose — the fuel of energy.[36]

Neuropsychologists Susan Resnick, Pauline Maki, and their colleagues, now at the National Institute of Aging, used PET scans to trace blood flow in the brains of thirty-two women, fifteen of whom were on estrogen and seventeen of whom were not, while they took tests of verbal and visual memory.* The estrogen users showed increased blood flow in the hippocampus and other brain regions involved in memory.[37] This evidence, which suggests a biological effect of estrogen on the brain, bolsters the behavioral evidence that comes from women's performance on memory tests. As Maki said to an interviewer from the American Psychological Association, "The fact that we found effects in the hippocampus makes it especially compelling."[38] The researchers concluded that

---

* PET studies and other physiological measures are costly and time-consuming, so researchers generally have to rely on small samples to test their early hypotheses. These researchers were trying to identify the biological underpinnings of cognitive skills or weaknesses.

the blood-flow findings suggest one route, though by no means the only one, by which estrogen protects against memory loss.

In sum, brain and animal studies support the conclusion that memory, neurotransmitter function, brain plasticity, blood flow, glucose metabolism, and neural protection are all enhanced by estrogen. Good news, but does it apply to women who take estrogen for longer than a short-lived lab study?

LESSONS FROM REAL LIFE

In 1952, in one of the earliest controlled studies of the effects of estrogen on women's cognitive functioning, Bettye McDonald Caldwell and Robert I. Watson tested twenty-eight women, average age seventy-five, who were living in a retirement home. They gave the women two well-established tests of verbal and other cognitive abilities — the Wechsler-Bellevue Intelligence Scale and the Wechsler Memory Scale — and then randomly assigned them to receive an injection of either estrogen or a placebo, administered once a week for a year, at which time the women were tested again. The results were impressive: The women who were taking estrogen during that year had a marked increase in their verbal IQ score on the intelligence and memory tests, whereas those given placebo showed a decrease on both measures of verbal ability. Another year later, following withdrawal of estrogen, the scores of all of these women had decreased back to their original baseline, indicating that estrogen's enhancement of memory occurred only while they were taking the hormone.[39]

In 1973, in another study of seventy-five-year-old women living

in a home for the aged, Herman Kantor and his colleagues randomly assigned twenty-five women to be given Premarin and
twenty-five to be given a placebo, daily, for three years. Every three
months, they compared the women's scores on the Hospital Adjust-
ment Scale, which measures behavior in three categories: commu-
nication and relationships, ability to take care of oneself, and work
activities. The scores of the women on Premarin increased steadily
for eighteen months and remained stable for the duration of the
study; the scores of those who were given the placebo decreased
steadily over time.[40] These well-controlled studies provided the first
compelling evidence that estrogen enhanced or maintained verbal
abilities, verbal memory, and aspects of social and physical functioning in women's everyday lives beyond the laboratory.

In the ensuing decades, the evidence from larger studies and
from other kinds of studies piled up, beginning with a groundbreaking 1988 study by psychologist Barbara Sherwin at McGill
University.[41] Sherwin, now retired, studied the effects of estrogen
on women's cognitive functioning for several decades, and three of
her early studies were especially influential. In the first, she worked
with women who had undergone surgery to remove the ovaries and
uterus, so their estrogen levels were very low. She randomly assigned
some of them to be given estrogen and the rest to receive a placebo,
and she immediately noticed a big difference. "Women who were
given a placebo after their surgery complained of not being able to
remember things, of having to make lists, which they never needed
to do in the past. They also had lower scores on tests of verbal
memory," she told a McGill reporter.[42] One test involves reading a
standard paragraph and then recalling the content, a measure of
short-term memory. Participants wait an hour or two, doing other

things, and then try to recall the paragraph again, a measure of longer-term memory. Women who received ERT after surgery performed better on tests of verbal memory and other cognitive functions than women who were given the placebo.

A few years later, Sherwin and her colleague Stuart Phillips conducted a study of otherwise healthy women who had had hysterectomies and removal of their ovaries for benign disease. The women took a battery of memory tests before surgery and again two months later after receiving injections of either estrogen or placebo. Those receiving estrogen either stayed at their pre-surgery cognitive level or, on one test, actually improved; those on placebo did worse on most of the verbal tests.[43]

And in a third study, Sherwin and Togas Tulandi, a research scientist and chief of McGill's department of obstetrics and gynecology, worked with nineteen premenopausal women who were being treated for benign uterine fibroids. (In doing medical research, large samples are nice, but you can't always get them, so you have to learn what you can from what's available. After all, you can't go into your local benign-uterine-fibroid bank and withdraw a thousand women.) The women took Lupron, which blocks the release of estrogen from the ovaries, every four weeks for twelve weeks. They were then randomly assigned to receive either add-back estrogen or placebo injections weekly for an additional eight weeks. When they were on Lupron, their scores on tests of verbal memory decreased from pretreatment to twelve weeks posttreatment, but those memory deficits were then reversed in the group that received estrogen. These findings "strongly suggest that estrogen serves to maintain verbal memory in women," the researchers concluded. Add-back estrogen regimens may be important for maintaining memory in women being treated with estrogen-suppressing medication as well as for women after menopause.[44]

And then there are the many studies that have followed women over even longer periods to see how they fared with and without estrogen.[45] Ming-Xin Tang, a biostatistician in the Alzheimer's Disease Research Center at Columbia University, and his colleagues followed 1,124 older women (their average age was seventy-four), initially free of Alzheimer's disease, who were taking part in a longitudinal study of aging and health in a New York City community. The researchers controlled for ethnicity, age, education, and APOE4 mutations. This was an observational study— meaning the women were not randomly assigned to take estrogen or a placebo—but the results were highly suggestive: Among women taking estrogen, the risk of developing Alzheimer's disease was significantly reduced by more than 60 percent; only 5.8 percent of the women on estrogen (9 of 156) developed the disease, as compared to 16.3 percent of the women who were not taking estrogen (158 of the 968). In addition, the age of onset of Alzheimer's disease occurred much later in women who were taking estrogen than in those who were not.[46] These results have been replicated in many different locations and around the world:

- United States: A study that followed 8,877 women in a retirement community for up to fourteen years found that estrogen users had a 45 percent decreased risk of developing Alzheimer's disease.[47]
- Italy: A population-based study of 2,816 women found that estrogen users had a 70 percent decreased risk of Alzheimer's disease.[48]

- Denmark: A major Danish randomized controlled trial, the Prospective Epidemiological Risk Factors Study, found that women randomly assigned to take HRT for two to three years had a 64 percent decreased risk of cognitive impairment five to fifteen years later as compared with those on placebo who had never taken hormones.[49]

Across these studies and others, the percentages of the decreased risk of dementia and Alzheimer's vary quite a bit, from 24 percent to 65 percent. But they all point in the same general direction: that estrogen helps. In 2000 and 2001, shortly before the first publication from the Women's Health Initiative, three large meta-analyses of existing studies concluded that, overall, hormone replacement therapy was associated with a 34 percent decreased risk of dementia and a nearly 40 percent decrease in the risk of Alzheimer's.[50]

DOES ESTROGEN INCREASE THE RISK OF STROKE?

Another form of cognitive impairment that is deeply frightening comes from having a stroke; the decreased blood supply to the brain results in the loss of functioning brain tissue. For decades, it has been known that premenopausal women have a lower risk of stroke than men of the same age and that after menopause, women's annual risk of stroke increases exponentially. That protection is also reduced among women who are deprived of estrogen before menopause.

We have noted that good observational studies often yield the same results as randomized controlled trials, but not always. Our goal for any given medical concern is to identify the overall picture that emerges from a variety of approaches, so let's see what that picture is for the risk of stroke for postmenopausal women who are taking HRT. Early observational studies produced a mixed bag of results. Some found that HRT decreased the risk of stroke;[51] some found that HRT had no effect at all;[52] and some found an increased risk.[53] One factor that might affect those outcomes is whether women have cardiovascular disease when they begin taking hormones. Fortunately, two randomized controlled trials helped answer that question. A study of 2,763 women with known heart disease whose mean age at the beginning of the study was sixty-seven and who were followed for an average of four years was published in 2001; it found no increased risk of stroke among the women randomly assigned to take HRT rather than the placebo.[54] That year, the results of a second randomized controlled trial of 664 women with a mean age of seventy-one at the outset of the study and a history of prior stroke was published; the women were followed for an average of nearly three years, and the investigators found no difference in the likelihood of having a stroke between the women treated with estrogen alone and those treated with placebo.[55]

And then, in 2004, Garnet Anderson and the rest of the small WHI steering committee announced that the estrogen-only arm of the study was being stopped because the use of estrogen increased the risk of nonfatal stroke by 12 per 10,000 women per year.[56] This was precisely what they had found in 2002, but apparently they didn't worry about it then; they waited two years to sound another alarm and set in motion another burst of "We're stopping the study!" headlines. Almost immediately, independent investigators published strong disagreements with this decision. Kate Maclaran and John Stevenson at the National Heart and Lung Institute, Imperial College London,[57] observed that the steering committee's concerns about stroke risks did not come at the recommendation of the WHI's own data safety and monitoring board. It was generated by the same inner group that had previously sounded the (false) alarm about hormones and breast cancer.

In fact, the WHI group had found no increase in any kind of serious stroke that led to incapacitation or death. They instead used an extremely broad definition of *stroke*—including transient, "subtle neurological deficits" that went away in a day or two with no aftermath.[58] Some epidemiologists argued that this small apparent increase was artificially introduced by a "detection bias"—that is, the fact that women on HRT, having been made so sensitive to possible adverse effects of hormones after 2002, were hyperalert to any neurological symptoms. (For example, if we told you that a tiny pimple on your forehead could indicate infection by a dangerous parasite, you'd become *very* attentive to tiny pimples.) A team of physicians led by George Mastorakos at National and Kapodistrian University of Athens reanalyzed the findings about the alleged risk of stroke. They published their results in the *Annals of the New York Academy of Sciences* under the title "Pitfalls of the Women's Health Initiative." Their reanalysis controlled for detection bias and the statistical manipulations that had appeared to indicate danger—and the supposed increased risk of stroke vanished.

Far from supporting the WHI's decision to stop the study, Mastorakos and his colleagues concluded this: "A closer look at the results of the WHI trial reveals that the use of HRT for 5 years should not be considered deleterious for the appearance of breast cancer, cardiovascular diseases, strokes, and pulmonary embolisms."

The regimen should be individualized for each patient, they added, and, in the interest of caution, women with a family history of breast cancer, diagnosed coronary disease, or a predisposition to deep vein thromboses should have more intense follow-up to look for worsening of any of these potential complications.[59]

Likewise, Stanley Birge, director of the Older Adult Health Center at Washington University School of Medicine in St. Louis, lamented the position of some medical societies that "persist in advising against the use of hormone therapy for the prevention of cardiovascular disease and osteoporosis" on the grounds that hormones increase the risk of stroke. That recommendation was ill-advised, he noted, because it was based on a misinterpretation of what the WHI study really found. The initial blip of increased risk among women most likely occurred because they were over sixty, overweight, hypertensive, and smokers, and thus probably had some degree of atherosclerotic disease to begin with. For women like them, Birge concluded, taking hormones might in fact create a slightly elevated risk during the first two or three years of use. But, he added, "there was no risk of adverse outcomes five or more years after initiation of hormone therapy and [in] younger women without [preexisting vascular] disease."[60]

One further note: A 2015 Cochrane analysis, headed by Henry Boardman of the department of cardiovascular medicine, University of Oxford, found no increased risk of stroke among women who started taking hormones before age sixty.[61] Cochrane reports are considered among the most reputable research findings in the medical literature, because they are meant to be impartial, independent assessments of the medical issue in question. (Archie Cochrane was a British physician who worked with Austin Bradford Hill and in 1972 published an influential book on the importance of evidence in medicine.) Drawing on a database of RCTs of women given hormone therapy or placebo and followed for at least six months—a total of nineteen trials with more than forty thousand women—they reported that women who started hormone therapy less than ten years after menopause had fewer deaths from cardiovascular causes and lower rates of coronary heart disease than women on placebo or no treatment. The Cochrane scientists found "no strong evidence of effect on risk of stroke in this group." Even among women who started taking hormones more than ten years after menopause, they found "high quality evidence that it had little effect on death or coronary heart disease between groups." Yet the Cochrane report issued one finding that is the reason that many doctors today still worry about the risk of stroke in all women on HRT; the investigators found "an increased risk of stroke among women who started taking hormones more than 10 years after menopause." How did that "increased risk of stroke" get in there? A Cochrane report is only as good as the data it is based on, and this finding was heavily influenced by the largest RCT in the literature, the Women's Health Initiative.

Reconciling the Evidence: The Optimal Window

Today, most of the leading scientists who study estrogen and brain function have refined the issue. Just as they concluded in assessing the risks and benefits of estrogen for heart disease, they suggest that the questions to ask are no longer *whether* estrogen helps but *whom* it helps and *when* it helps.

We have already mentioned one such investigator, Roberta Diaz

Brinton, who summarized her view this way: For the most part, women who begin estrogen or HRT at the time of menopause reduce their risk of getting many forms of dementia, including Alzheimer's. But studies of women who are given estrogen as a treatment—once they have already developed a degree of dementia—have mixed results. For example, in a randomized double-blind clinical trial of estrogen given to female Alzheimer's patients over age seventy-two, estrogen produced a modest improvement in the short term (two months) but a worsening of the disease in the long term (twelve months). Other studies have gotten similar results. A review of the medical records of fifty-five hundred patients who were followed at Kaiser Permanente found that women who had started taking hormones around menopause had a 26 percent decreased risk of subsequent dementia, but those who started hormones many years after menopause had a 48 percent increased risk.[62] Brinton concluded that "as the continuum of neurological health progresses from healthy to unhealthy, so too do the benefits of estrogen or hormone therapy. If neurons are healthy at the time of estrogen exposure, their response to estrogen is beneficial for both neurological function and survival."[63] But if those neurons are not healthy when a woman starts estrogen or if she begins taking HRT ten or more years after menopause, estrogen may, over time, make her condition worse.

Barbara Sherwin concluded too that the evidence from basic neuroscience, from animal studies, and from human studies provided a strong case for a "critical window of opportunity." In a paper for the Canadian Consensus on Menopause and Osteoporosis, she wrote: "Estrogen replacement prevents deterioration of aspects of cognition in older women that occurs with normal aging.

There is also compelling evidence that ERT prevents or delays the onset of Alzheimer's disease in women who are at risk for genetic or environmental reasons."[64] But, she added, there is no evidence that estrogen can slow or alleviate the disease once a woman has been diagnosed with it. Women who start estrogen when menopause begins, Sherwin said, thereby "seamlessly extending" the number of years their brains are exposed to it, will likely have less cognitive decline as they get older. Once they stopped taking HRT or ERT, however, it was not clear whether estrogen's protective benefits would continue into very old age; there were just not enough good studies done with women that extended for thirty years after menopause to know for sure, nor was such a large RCT ever likely to be done. Sherwin hoped that animal studies and "creative ways of asking this question in humans will provide some answers in the future."[65]

There currently are some promising studies indicating that for estrogen to be maximally effective in reducing the risk of Alzheimer's, it needs to be taken for at least ten years.[66] Pauline Maki has also proposed the window-of-opportunity hypothesis to reconcile the WHI's claims with the many studies that contradict it. Studies that reported an improvement in cognitive function, she observed, had assessed women who received estrogen at the time of menopause, whereas those studies that reported no improvement, such as the Women's Health Initiative, involved women who started HRT many years after menopause. Women who started HRT somewhere between the ages of fifty and their early sixties had the greatest benefit; for women who began HRT in their sixties, hormones neither increased nor decreased their risk of Alzheimer's. A study whose name is hard to forget—the REMEMBER study (from Research into Memory, Brain Function and Estrogen Replacement)—likewise found that the timing of hormone therapy for women over age sixty was important in determining whether estrogen would help their later cognitive abilities.[67]

What About the Alternatives?

Most Americans don't like the idea that there are no drugs available to slow, let alone cure, Alzheimer's and other dementias, and this discomfort makes them vulnerable to the simplistic allures of untested products and promises. In 2017, the Federal Trade Commission filed a complaint against the makers of a bestselling supplement called Prevagen, claiming the company was falsely advertising it as a memory booster that gets "into the brain" and improves cognition. Prevagen, reportedly made from a protein in jellyfish, has been heavily marketed with commercials on CNN, Fox News, NBC, and elsewhere, mostly on the grounds that it is a bestselling product. "The marketers of Prevagen preyed on the fears of older consumers experiencing age-related memory loss," said the director of the FTC's Bureau of Consumer Protection. "But one critical thing these marketers forgot is that their claims need to be backed up by real scientific evidence."[68] There is none. (The government's case was dismissed by the trial court but is presently on appeal.)

The most widely prescribed drugs for Alzheimer's symptoms, Aricept and Remeron, allow patients, physicians, and family members the comfort of thinking that *something* is being done to help, but, sadly, those somethings are often no better than nothing, and they're a lot more costly. What, then, might help? Popular writers advise all kinds of benign interventions: eating a diet rich in anti-oxidants, reducing stress, engaging in stimulating mental activities like crossword puzzles, and exercising regularly. On the Mayo Clinic website, you'll find more of this optimistic all-purpose advice: "Regular exercise and a walking program have been found to prevent cognitive decline." That adviser apparently didn't speak to another physician on the website who answered the question "Are there any proven Alzheimer's prevention strategies?" with "Not yet."[69] While acknowledging that "more research is needed" before any advice could be considered a proven strategy, he added the usual recommendations to lead a healthy lifestyle: Get regular physical activity, preferably aerobic. Eat a healthy Mediterranean diet that is rich in vegetables and olive oil. Keep your brain active (all those crossword puzzles). Don't smoke. Control your blood pressure and cholesterol. Use your thinking skills. ("Use it or lose it" is a popular refrain, although gerontologists often gloomily add, "If you've lost it, you can't use it.")

We have no objection to healthy diets, olive oil, and exercise, mental and physical. But as interventions that might truly have a beneficial effect on delaying or averting cognitive decline and dementia in a woman's later years, compared to estrogen, they don't do much.

Nowadays people are exhorted to regard the brain as just another muscle, one that can be exercised to keep it from getting flabby and plump. Memory exercises are today's mental weights; accordingly, numerous online programs are available to help people strengthen working memory, one of the mental systems responsible for storing and manipulating information. Working-memory training originated in 1999, when cognitive neuroscientist Torkel Klingberg created a computer program designed to help children with ADHD learn to focus. By 2001, he launched his company, Cogmed, and initial studies of children with attention deficit problems were promising. Naturally, that early success led to the hope that it would help people with other impairments of working memory—everything from mild learning difficulties to strokes and other forms of brain damage—improve their reasoning, everyday lapses of attention, and recall.

We're unhappy that we don't have happier news. Monica Melby-Lervåg, in the department of special needs education at the University of Oslo, and her colleagues Thomas S. Redick and Charles Hulme published a meta-analysis of working-memory training studies—87 publications involving 145 experimental comparisons.[70] All of the studies had a pretest/posttest method and a control group and were designed to see whether working-memory training helped short-term recall and if it transferred to other measures of mental ability. Typically, right after training, people improved on measures of near transfer—that is, doing what they had just learned to do. Practice doing puzzles and you get better at doing puzzles. Unfortunately, for measures of far transfer (nonverbal ability, verbal ability, word decoding, reading comprehension, and arithmetic), the researchers found "no convincing evidence of any reliable improvements when working-memory training was compared with a treated control condition.... Working-memory training programs appear to produce short-term, specific training effects that do not generalize to measures of 'real-world' cognitive skills." Damn.

At the Georgia Institute of Technology, memory scientist Randall W. Engel and his lab have found the same thing. In their own meta-analytic review, they concluded that "there is no good evidence that working-memory training improves intelligence test scores or other measures of 'real-world' cognitive skills."[71] Thomas Redick, another cognitive psychologist in their lab, took a close look at five studies that claimed to have demonstrated benefits of working-memory training; where benefits occurred right after the intervention, they were gone in a few months.[72] These findings were extended and confirmed in a 2016 meta-analysis of studies of "brain-training programs" that specifically focused on whether using cognitive tasks or games enhanced performance on other tasks.[73] Regrettably, they did not.

Well, then, forget mental training; how about brain training? Transcranial direct-current stimulation (tDCS)—a noninvasive technique that applies electric current to areas of the brain—is growing in popularity for treating a variety of problems and disorders, from reducing depression to improving cognitive abilities. But researchers at the Karolinska Institute in Stockholm found that applying tDCS to the brains of older people while they were immersed in working-memory training did not do much of anything for them. They enrolled 123 healthy adults between the ages of sixty-five and seventy-five in a four-week training program. Everyone took a battery of cognitive tests at the beginning of the study and again at the end. Some participants received twenty-five minutes of tDCS to an area of the prefrontal cortex that plays a central role in working memory; others were led to believe they were receiving twenty-five minutes of current when in reality the current was active for only thirty seconds. The former group showed no improvement in cognitive skills over their peers who got the sham treatment. When the researchers pooled the data from this study with findings from six other studies, they again found no evidence of any additional benefit from working-memory training that was combined with tDCS.

The hope that tDCS would be a safe and effective way to improve cognitive function, the researchers concluded, "has been as seductive to the research community as it has been to the media. A growing number of people in the general public, presumably inspired by such uninhibited optimism, are now using tDCS to perform better at work or in online gaming, and online communities offer advice on the purchase, fabrication, and use of tDCS devices. Unsurprisingly, commercial exploitation is rapidly being developed to meet this new public demand for cognitive enhancement via tDCS, often without a single human trial to support the sellers' or manufacturers' claims."[74]

If mental exercises don't help memory and other cognitive abilities, how about physical exercise, which is widely believed to be an effective preventive for dementia? Notice the waffling tone in the Mayo Clinic's advice: "More research is needed to know to what degree adding physical activity improves memory or slows the progression of cognitive decline. Nonetheless, regular exercise is important to stay physically and mentally fit." Translation: Exercise is good, and it seems logical that it would slow the progression of cognitive decline and do other good things for your brain, but we don't yet know how much exercise or what kind is helpful. Still, do it anyway.

We agree. But Carol, who is a devotee of Pilates, weights, and walking and who is well past her window of opportunity for HRT, dispatched her medical co-author to scour the literature for evidence that exercise would keep her brain from declining any more than it has. There are literally hundreds of published papers that claim to show that exercise helps forestall cognitive decline, but even the ten best ones disintegrate under close inspection. Some authors cite others' claims, not their own original research. Some studies rely on participants' memories of how much exercise they think they did—or remember thinking they did—years earlier, but self-reporting is notoriously unreliable. Some studies use measures of exercise that vary widely in both frequency (from one hour a week to one hour or more daily) and degree of intensity (from just getting out of your chair to vigorous walking or running). Or exercise is confounded with other risk factors, notably obesity, diabetes, lower education, and depression. And if exercise is difficult to measure accurately in these studies, so is cognitive decline; the measurements range from mild to severe. These complexities do not stop the writers of what we call "if-only" headlines, such as this one from the British paper the *Telegraph* purporting to summarize a new study: "One Hour of Exercise a Week 'Can Halve Dementia Risk.'"[75] If only!

But because animal studies show that exercise does have neurological and vascular benefits in the brain, the effort to link those changes to cognitive abilities continues. A 2014 meta-analysis of forty-seven longitudinal studies that tracked the effects of physical activity on cognitive decline and dementia found that people with "higher levels of physical activity, when compared to those with lower levels, are at reduced risk of cognitive decline." Overall, what was that reduced risk? Only 18 percent. (Not to be sneezed at, though—get out of that chair.) Unfortunately, the better the study, the weaker the finding.[76]

More recently, in the January 2018 *Annals of Internal Medicine*, Michelle Brasure and her colleagues at the University of Minnesota and Brown University reviewed thirty-two trials assessing the effectiveness of physical activity in slowing cognitive decline and delaying the onset of cognitive impairment and dementia among healthy adults. "The evidence was insufficient to draw conclusions about the effectiveness of aerobic training, resistance training, or tai chi for improving cognition," the researchers concluded. Some interventions were helpful, but "evidence regarding effects on dementia prevention was insufficient for all physical activity interventions."[77]

THE TAKE-HOME

When Barbara Sherwin launched what would be her decades-long work on menopause, hormones, and memory, she feared the media might turn her findings into simplistic advice or, worse, use them to foster the misogynistic view of postmenopausal women's reduced cognitive abilities. Still, as she told a reporter at her home university of McGill, her goal has always been to help women live as enjoyably and productively as possible, and so she has little patience for those who dismiss HRT because it is "unnatural." "What's not natural is to live to 80," she said. Women live anywhere from one-third to one-half of their lives after menopause, and if estrogen helps cognition and staves off Alzheimer's, that is crucial information. But

Sherwin has never been a "feminine forever" advocate. "Enhancing quality of life," she said, "is not the same as getting rid of the phenomenon of aging."[78]

So, to review: There are good reasons to believe that estrogen helps maintain cognitive abilities, prevents both cardiovascular disease (as we saw in chapter 3) and stroke, and reduces the risk of Alzheimer's disease.

- Estrogen stimulates the growth of nerve cells, regenerates axons, and decreases the nerve-cell death that happens in Alzheimer's. It makes brain cells more responsive to the effects of nerve growth factor and reduces the production of substances associated with Alzheimer's, such as beta amyloid and tau protein.
- Estrogen reduces levels of vasoconstrictors, substances that narrow the arteries; increases levels of vasodilators, substances that expand them; increases cerebral blood flow; and inhibits inflammatory substances that are involved in the early stages of atherosclerosis.[79]
- Estrogen enhances the ability of neurons to survive a variety of physiological insults, such as disease and brain injury.
- The Women's Health Initiative did not find an increased risk of dementia or cognitive impairment in women on estrogen only. The risk was slightly increased among women on HRT, but only if they had preexisting cognitive impairments or were starting hormones long past menopause (over age seventy-five).
- The Women's Health Initiative did not find that estrogen increased the risk of stroke in younger women entering

menopause who were in good vascular health. There was an increased risk in women who were over sixty, overweight, hypertensive, and smokers, and thus probably had some degree of atherosclerotic disease to begin with.

- Just as with estrogen's benefits for heart and bones, there does seem to be a window of opportunity for estrogen to have a long-standing cognitive benefit: the decade following the onset of menopause. If estrogen is begun after around age sixty or many years after menopause begins, it may be ineffective and possibly risky.

Recently, Av received yet another frustrated, angry message from a former patient we'll call Linda. Nearly twenty-five years ago, she had an invasive breast cancer that was greater than two centimeters; her lymph nodes were negative for cancer, and she was treated with a lumpectomy, radiation, and chemotherapy. She has been on Premarin and progesterone ever since and has had no evidence of recurrence in all those years. Having moved out of state, she wrote to Av: "I'm still taking HRT and would appreciate getting a copy of your pertinent research on it because I have to beg the doctors to approve it or prescribe it. I once stopped it, but within two or three weeks I became very old and couldn't remember a thing. I was in a meeting and at some point I realized I had just asked the same question for the third time. Imagine my embarrassment! I've never stopped [HRT] again."

And so Av sent her some "pertinent research," a few papers based on the Women's Health Initiative itself. The WHI, as usual, had made a lot of noise about HRT's harms (dementia! stroke!) but buried HRT's benefits. Av dug through their reports and pulled out a plum: The WHI's own data showed that women who had taken hormones prior to entering the study, and therefore closer to the time of menopause, were less likely to develop all forms of dementia, including Alzheimer's, during the clinical trial. They had a reduction of risk of 50 percent compared to nonusers.[80] We hope that information persuaded Linda's doctor, as, along with decades of supporting research, it has persuaded us.

6

Can Breast Cancer Survivors Take Estrogen?

Thus far, we have been addressing concerns that many healthy women have: Will taking hormones increase the risk of breast cancer? Will they alleviate menopausal symptoms? How might they reduce the risk of serious diseases? In this chapter, Avrum will make a counterintuitive but well-supported claim that even among women who have had breast cancer, HRT is a reasonable option and provides the benefits already discussed in this book. It's Av's story, so he will tell it from his point of view.

*   *   *

Several years ago, I was called to be an expert witness for the prosecution in a medical malpractice case involving a patient with lung cancer. The diagnosis had been delayed for over a year because the radiologist had missed an abnormality on the patient's chest X-ray.

The tumor, which could have been surgically removed a year earlier, was now inoperable.

I clearly remember being cross-examined by the attorney for the defense. He held up a large, weighty textbook, *Cancer: Principles and Practice of Oncology,* and asked: "Dr. Bluming, isn't it true that this textbook is called the bible of cancer medicine?" I told him I was thoroughly familiar with the textbook, which was highly respected in my field, but that no book of medicine is a bible. He handed it to me and asked me to open it to a particular page and read a marked paragraph about lung cancer. The paragraph asserted that since the prognosis in lung cancer was invariably fatal, early diagnosis was of no benefit to the patient. The attorney asked for my response. "There is a reference in this paragraph to a specific article," I said, "which, by a fortunate coincidence, I have brought to the trial." I read the article for the court. It stated that early diagnosis and treatment in that type of lung cancer would greatly improve the chance for cure. The textbook author had misquoted the article. The cancer bible was fallible.

I haven't been that lucky with any specific reference since, one that clarifies an issue and its resolution in one shot. On the contrary, I am well aware that in the practice of medicine, physicians can invariably find references to support almost any opinion. I have attended many medical conferences that degenerated into an exercise of dueling references, with each side citing only those articles that supported its position. That is why I have made every effort to seek not only the studies that support my opinions but also the studies that contest them. When you are a physician, the question of the evidence you rely on to make a decision about an intervention or treatment becomes more than an academic debate at a conference or in a journal; your patients' well-being, health, and often lives depend on the advice you offer and the decisions you make. You therefore want the very best evidence to guide your practice, while also leaving room for your years of experience and clinical judgment.

Yet sometimes there isn't a good reference to guide you; sometimes there are no clear answers. In my lifetime in oncology—and I became an oncologist before the specialty was even named—two clinical decisions were of paramount personal importance to me: whether or not to endorse the movement away from radical mastectomy in favor of the less invasive lumpectomy and whether or not to prescribe HRT for patients whom I had treated for breast cancer.

In the mid-1970s, I moved from an academic appointment in Boston to the private practice of medical oncology in Southern California. At that time, several clinical investigators around the world were exploring lumpectomy followed by radiotherapy as an alternative to traditional mastectomy for the treatment of newly diagnosed breast cancer. This was a dramatic departure from standard medical practice, and many surgeons reacted with understandable resistance. "The only way to reduce the risk of recurrence is to remove the breast and as much adjacent tissue as possible," many said, "and now you are telling me to remove only the lump? Anything less than total mastectomy would be malpractice." At my hospital, the chief of surgery would go from operating room to operating room asking the surgeons what surgery they were performing. When the surgeon replied, "A mastectomy," he would shout, "Way to go!"

My fellow Los Angeles oncologists strongly advised me not to pursue the issue of lumpectomy and not to recommend it to my patients. I would be dependent on surgical referrals to help build my practice, they said, and mastectomy was bread-and-butter surgery for practicing surgeons. By trying to alter the paradigm of how breast cancer should be treated, I would turn off referrals from these necessary sources. Since all of my medical training had been done back east, I had no hospital or university contacts that might supplement patient referrals to my new oncology practice. I thanked my new colleagues, but I did not follow their advice. I decided on a plan of cooperation and persuasion instead of an adversarial battle.

As chair of the professional educational committee of the American Cancer Society for the San Fernando Valley chapter, then the second largest in the nation, I invited Sam Hellman, a professor and chair of the department of radiation therapy at Harvard Medical School and one of the early pioneers of lumpectomy research, to speak to a large audience of physicians and surgeons. His data were powerful and persuasive, and I could see that the edges of the iceberg of doubt and opposition in that room were melting. But it took the surgeons' own experiences to fully persuade them. Mike Drickman, one of the first surgeons in Los Angeles to switch to lumpectomy, told me that after he did his first one, "I was so overwhelmed by the gratitude of the patient that whenever I can, I offer lumpectomy as the first option to all my breast cancer patients who need surgery."

To further my collaborative approach, I invited physicians across specialties to begin a community-wide study in which they would assemble data on their patients and then chart what happened after lumpectomy. The community team consisted of eight medical oncologists, seventeen breast surgeons, seven radiation therapists, and seven pathologists, and when I wrote up the results of our study for the *Annals of Surgery,* I listed all thirty-nine of us as co-authors. The editor, who must have been amused by all those names marching across the page, told me I could have only three. But I was grateful for, and proud of, my colleagues for their open-minded yet critical review of emerging data in this field, so I replied that I wanted all of those names not only printed but also identified by specialty. By this, I hoped to recognize their willingness to work across different areas of expertise, highlight the diversity of perspectives they brought to the research, and encourage further community collaborations of this kind. The editor agreed.[1] Referrals to my practice did not suffer, and the Los Angeles community became one of the earliest adopters of this new treatment for primary breast cancer.

As a physician, I rely on the medical literature to inform me of what the empirical evidence shows, but I also depend on other physicians' clinical experience. The greatest challenge in the practice of oncology is finding the best approach to a medical problem at the time you need it, and that approach might not yet have been published. Many years ago, I was asked to see a sixteen-year-old boy with newly diagnosed Ewing's sarcoma of a rib. At that time, the cure rate for this disease was close to zero, information ignored by his grandmother, who said to me, "Dr. Bluming, I did not survive Auschwitz to watch my grandson die of cancer."

I reviewed the world literature and found no treatment that had been successful. I consulted Mark Nesbitt, chair of the National Ewing's Cooperative Group, who had no therapeutic suggestions. I consulted Gus Higgins, the principal investigator of the children's Cancer Study Group in Los Angeles; he didn't have any promising leads either. I consulted Audrey Evans, a leading medical oncologist at Children's Hospital in Philadelphia; she did have a protocol for treatment but little evidence of its success. I eventually found Gerald Rosen, a pediatric oncologist at Memorial Sloan Kettering Cancer Center in New York. He had treated more than fifty young patients with Ewing's sarcoma using a combination of intensive chemotherapy drugs, and he was having remarkable success. In the overwhelming majority of his patients, he told me, the cancer had disappeared and not returned, even after several years. He had not yet published the results of his intensive regimen; it would be another year before he did. But I was persuaded by the fact that he had more experience with this rare tumor than anyone else, and he was getting encouraging results. I used his regimen with my patient. That was more than twenty-five years ago, and that teenager is now a healthy middle-aged man.

The practice of oncology thus requires a constant dance between what we know and what we must learn; perhaps that's why we say that surgeons *perform* surgery but physicians *practice* medicine.

In the early 1990s, my wife and many of my other breast cancer patients began asking me if they could take HRT. They wanted to relieve the severe menopause-associated symptoms that were impairing the quality of their lives, but they were afraid of fueling a recurrence of the breast cancer. I was understandably apprehensive. So were they. It seemed a no-brainer. Why would I even consider administering ERT or HRT to women with a history of breast cancer? What if the cancer returned? What if I were responsible for the death of a patient who, without my well-intentioned help, might have remained cured? I felt pangs of empathy for the surgeons who could not give up doing radical mastectomies, unable to shake the fear that it would put their patients at greater risk of recurrence. Nonetheless, the frequent requests from my patients for something to alleviate their distress motivated me to seek new answers.

STEP ONE: LOOKING FOR CLUES

In those days, some twenty-five years ago, we didn't have enough good data on the consequences of giving HRT to breast cancer survivors for oncologists to say for sure that it was harmful, beneficial, or neither. Like the experts I consulted for Ewing's sarcoma, physicians who were doing the best they could with limited research to guide them, some oncologists were prescribing hormones for their breast cancer patients, but they did so with varying degrees of follow-up and no consistent treatment protocol.

So I had to look for clues in related conditions. Where might I see whether estrogen increased the risk of recurrence in women who had had breast cancer? I started by evaluating the then-common belief that premenopausal breast cancer survivors should have their ovaries removed as a precaution. Because the ovaries produce estrogen, and because estrogen was "known" to cause breast cancer, that intervention made sense. But it was wrong. William Creasman, a gynecologist-oncologist at the Medical University of South Carolina, observed that prospective randomized studies showed that this intervention had no benefit in reducing the risk of recurrence of cancer or in prolonging a woman's survival, which is why it is no longer done (though, as with all procedures in medicine, there are a few diehards who still believe it is beneficial). "Thus, estrogen appears to be all right in the premenopausal breast cancer patient," he wrote, "but, for some reason, estrogen administration to the postmenopausal patient is not. Why?"[2]

Next, because estrogen and progesterone levels soar during pregnancy, I looked at what research had to say about women who become pregnant after having breast cancer. In 1991, Mitchell Gail and Jacques Benichou of the National Cancer Institute observed that because pregnancy markedly elevates a woman's levels of estrogen and progesterone, women who get pregnant when they are young and then have many children should have the highest risk of developing breast cancer. Then they added, "And, of course, the converse is the case."[3] *Of course* the converse is the case? Again, the evidence was counterintuitive.

As long ago as 1970, a World Health Organization report had shown that women who completed a full-term pregnancy before age twenty had one-third the usual risk of later developing breast cancer.[4] Why, then, would breast cancer patients be at risk of a recurrence if they got pregnant? It turns out they aren't. In 1989, Alan Wile, a surgeon, and Philip DiSaia, chair of the division of gynecologic oncology, both at the University of California, Irvine, reported that pregnancy, either during or after treatment for breast cancer, had no negative effect on prognosis. (In 2017, that finding was replicated in an international study led by oncologist Matteo Lambertini of the Institut Jules Bordet in Brussels.[5]) Wile and DiSaia also noted that there was no benefit in removing their patients' ovaries and that as long as patients were informed "that there is no evidence that estrogen has an adverse effect upon established breast cancer," they felt it was appropriate to let them take HRT to alleviate menopausal symptoms and improve well-being.[6]

Thus far, I was finding that neither lowering estrogen levels (by removing ovaries) nor raising estrogen levels (becoming pregnant) increased the recurrence of breast cancer. And, as we reported in chapter 1, there was already considerable historical evidence of estrogen's benefits. In 1966, Charles Huggins was awarded the Nobel Prize for showing that hormones could control the spread of some cancers. Using a sample of rats that had been given a carcinogen that produces breast cancer, he found that giving rats high levels of estradiol and progesterone for thirty days inhibited the emergence of breast cancers and that only one week of treatment was enough to demonstrate this effect.[7] It took years before Huggins's Nobel Prize–worthy findings were applied to women, but the results were promising. I noted with interest three studies published in the 1980s, conducted by researchers in Europe and England:

— Torben Palshof, an oncologist at University Hospital Gentofte in Copenhagen, and his colleagues reported on 332 patients with breast cancer who, after surgery and radiation, were randomly assigned to be given DES (diethylstilbestrol, a form of estrogen), tamoxifen, or placebo for two years. Five years later, at follow-up, the women receiving DES had the lowest rate of cancer recurrence, similar to the rate of women given tamoxifen, and the women on the placebo had a significantly higher recurrence rate. When Palshof conducted another follow-up in 1985, the results were unchanged.[8]

— Louk V.A.M. Beex, an oncologist at St. Radboud University Hospital in Nijmegen, the Netherlands, and his colleagues randomized sixty-three postmenopausal women with advanced breast cancer to receive tamoxifen or estrogen to see how their tumors responded. Although tamoxifen was believed to block estrogen and therefore be more beneficial, they found that although the tumors in 33 percent of the patients on tamoxifen shrank, surprisingly so did those of 31 percent of patients on estrogen.[9]

—Basil Stoll, a British endocrinologist who wrote an early textbook on hormonal management in patients with breast cancer, reported that he had administered estrogen and progesterone to sixty-five postmenopausal women with advanced breast cancer and found that after six months of treatment, 22 percent of the women showed a regression of the cancer.[10]

I also found numerous oncologists risking the disagreement and even outright opprobrium of colleagues and saying that the time was right for research on giving HRT to breast cancer survivors. For example, Michael Baum, who was then chair of the Breast Cancer Trials Coordinating Committee in London and a member of the academic department of surgery at the Royal Marsden Hospital, wrote, "I find it intolerable that we should have to carry on in ignorance about the benefits and risks of prescribing hormone replacement therapy to women who have had breast cancer. There are occasions when the indications for hormone replacement therapy must take precedence over any theoretical objections. It is clearly inhumane when a woman who is already having to cope with the physical and psychological burden of breast cancer is then expected to accept, without relief, some of the serious effects of the menopause, which can include severe depression."[11]

With this empirical and clinical grounding, I felt ready to launch a study in which breast cancer survivors who were in complete remission following initial treatment but who were suffering from menopausal symptoms would be given HRT. They would be followed over time to see if HRT increased the risk of the breast cancer's return.[12]

Step Two: Dealing with the FDA

I began this effort by discussing my research proposal with most of the medical oncologists in the Los Angeles area as well as with gynecologists and primary-care physicians. Their participation was crucial in giving me critical evaluations of the data I would be collecting and the assumptions I was making, and many of them added their own patients to the study once it was under way.

All of those I consulted supported going ahead with the study, but several expressed one major reservation: a fear of legal culpability if a woman in the study had a recurrence. I therefore contacted Ned Good, the president of the California Bar Association, who told me that anybody can sue anybody for anything, and we would have no guaranteed protection from a lawsuit. However, he added, the best proactive defense would be to ensure that every patient understood the risks entailed in joining the study and to have that understanding confirmed with a signed informed-consent form. Done.

I then called the Food and Drug Administration, told them what I was planning to do, and asked whether I needed FDA approval to proceed. They said that if I called what I was doing a *treatment,* FDA approval was unnecessary; some physicians, they were aware, were already administering HRT to breast cancer survivors without FDA approval. If, however, I wished to call what I was proposing a *study,* then I was advised to submit a full protocol to the FDA, with details of the methods, goals, rationale, and references from the medical literature. That took a little longer, but it was done.

Six weeks after receiving my proposal, a doctor at the FDA called to tell me that it had been put on a clinical hold, primarily because the FDA felt that the study would place women at an increased risk of breast cancer recurrence.

"Has anyone there actually read my full proposal?" I asked him. "The part where I describe the studies indicating that estrogen is safer than most physicians realize, even for breast cancer survivors?"

"Don't shoot me," he said. "I'm just the messenger."

I asked to speak to someone who had decision-making ability, and, instead of having a second phone conversation, I was invited to testify before an FDA subcommittee in Rockville, Maryland, on Valentine's Day 1992. Before leaving, I met with Alan Wile, one of the breast cancer investigators who I knew had called for such research. We rehearsed a joint presentation. I offered to coordinate a pilot study for three hundred women, and Alan, speaking for his department at UC Irvine, agreed that if we found no increased risk of breast cancer recurrence in the pilot study, his university would commit to a long-term, double-blind, randomized study of this issue with a population of five thousand postmenopausal women.

We delivered our presentations at the committee meeting, which was open to the public. One women's health activist implored the panel to deny our proposal, arguing that giving estrogen to women who had had breast cancer was tantamount to giving them a "poison valentine." But at the end of the meeting, the female chair of the committee said she thought it would be unethical *not* to do this study. On the flight home, Alan cautioned me not to think our study had been approved.

"It sounded like approval to me," I said.

"Just wait," he advised. Several weeks later, the FDA let us know that although they had approved the study in principle, they objected to the details I had specified for a small pilot study. The only proposal they would approve, they said, would be for a prospective double-blind randomized trial of six thousand to eight thousand women. I protested this decision because, as the committee members were aware, some breast cancer survivors were already being treated with HRT in pockets around the country, with no attempt to collect relevant data. We would be collecting follow-up data on our treated patients rather than allowing their results to be lost. If we found we were harming them, surely, we felt, it would be preferable to discover this in a small pilot study rather than a large one.

"Sorry," the FDA said (in effect). "The big study or none."

Undeterred, I returned to the FDA on my own dime, and, to its credit, the FDA organized another committee meeting to hear me out. Before the formal discussion began, some of the physicians on the committee asked me questions that felt surreal.

"Why don't you do a different study?" one male doctor asked. "Why are you fixated on doing this particular one?"

"I *do* other studies," I said. "However, because the evidence persuades me that we have been wrong about estrogen's harms, and because we don't know enough about giving estrogen to breast cancer survivors, I feel this study is important."

"Why do you even need to do this study?" asked a female physician. "Isn't it true that most of your patients are going to die anyway?"

"I'm sorry, but you are misinformed," I told her. "The current cure rate for early breast cancer is now running higher than eighty-five percent."

"Perhaps I should refresh my knowledge on the subject," she said.

"That would be good," I agreed.

During the several-hour committee meeting that followed, I was unable to convince any member that the pilot study I proposed was worth doing before undertaking a larger study of several thousand women. As I was leaving, I asked the chair what would happen if I returned to my community and proceeded with the study I wanted to do. "We can't tell you how to practice medicine, Dr. Bluming," he said. "I hope you have found our comments to be beneficial." I thanked them for taking the time to meet with me but told them I found their comments to be of no help. I returned to Los Angeles to run the study.

Step Three: Doing the Pilot Study

At least the FDA had unanimously concurred that my proposed research was ethical. "We agree," they (eventually) wrote in *JAMA,* "that clinical trials are needed to address this issue [of HRT for breast cancer patients] and wish to note that on February 14, 1992, the Division of Metabolism and Endocrine Drug Products of the FDA convened its Fertility and Maternal Health Drugs Advisory Committee for public discussion of the issues involved. During the proceedings, the committee voted unanimously yes to the question: is it ethical to conduct well-designed clinical trials of hormone replacement therapy in women who have been treated for breast cancer, when a primary outcome of interest will be to ascertain whether the treatment causes breast cancer recurrence?"[13]

As soon as I returned home, I addressed the annual meeting of the Los Angeles ob-gyn society and officially launched the pilot study of the effects of hormone replacement on breast cancer survivors. I made sure that every woman understood the potential benefits and risks of the medication, as well as the purpose of the study. And I made sure that the "caution statement" from the FDA was clearly positioned in the informed-consent form:

> Although the FDA has endorsed the rationale for testing the potential benefits and risks of hormone replacement therapy in women with a history of treated breast cancer, the FDA committee responsible for reviewing this particular study feels that no meaningful data will be provided due to the small number of patients to be evaluated (300) and the absence of a randomized group of comparable women who will receive no hormone replacement therapy. The FDA committee raised the concern that any results from so small a study population on non-randomized patients might be overinterpreted to yield conclusions of benefit or risk that were premature or inaccurate.

All of the women gave their consent. Because I knew that a symptomatic woman would know whether or not she was receiving estrogen within a few days — after all, these women wanted to take HRT precisely to alleviate menopausal symptoms — there was no placebo control group. (This problem — of participants in any study knowing whether they are getting the real drug or a placebo — afflicts much research, even gold-standard RCTs and the Women's Health Initiative. In studies of menopausal symptoms, a woman will know soon enough what she's taking.) I did, however, compare the hormone-treated group with women who had been diagnosed with the same stage of breast cancer, who had been treated the same way over the same period, and who lived in the same community. If I were to discover an unanticipated risk of recurrence among my patients or found any published paper demonstrating an increased risk—that is, any evidence that giving my patients HRT was pouring fuel on a fire—I would halt the study immediately.

I began this work in 1992, and for the next fourteen years I published an annual update on the participants, with 100 percent follow-up on the 248 women who were enrolled over time. Even the women who had moved out of state during those years provided me with medical information on how they were doing.[14] My goal was to determine whether these women showed an increased incidence of recurrence of breast cancer in the same breast, developed cancer in the other breast, or developed breast cancer metastases elsewhere in the body.

And this is what I found: they did not. Yes, a few of these women had a recurrence of breast cancer, but not at a rate higher than the comparable women who were not on HRT.

In 1997, I was invited to present the five-year results of our study to eighty-five hundred oncologists at the American Society of Clinical Oncology's annual conference in Denver. The presentation preceding mine was given by a physician from the National Cancer Institute. He told the crowd that "the NCI is not sponsoring HRT symptom relief or disease prevention studies in breast cancer survivors." Based on the computer models, he concluded,

"Hormone replacement therapy can only harm breast cancer survivors."

I remember thinking I would probably be stoned for presenting my small pilot study from a community in Southern California after this preemptive condemnation by a spokesperson from the National Cancer Institute. But that's not the way it turned out. After the presentation, all the questions and comments from this large, international audience of leading oncologists and researchers were positive. In contrast, the audience's response to the NCI presentation was uniformly negative.

"Don't shoot me," the NCI guy said. "I'm only the messenger."

The following year, 1998, the FDA informed me that the clinical hold that had been placed on my study six years earlier—the study I had continued, reported on annually, and presented at the 1997 ASCO annual meeting—was being lifted.

This response from ASCO and the FDA was, of course, gratifying. But it was even more gratifying to realize that my study was now part of a larger phenomenon—the medical establishment's resistance to treating breast cancer patients with HRT was melting, just as its resistance to lumpectomy had melted a decade before.* In a thorough review of the research up to 1994, Melody Cobleigh, a medical oncologist at Rush–Presbyterian–St. Luke's Medical Center in Chicago, and her colleagues in the Breast Cancer Committees of the Eastern Cooperative Oncology Group wrote: "A major

---

* The recent rise in mastectomies that we noted in the introduction is a result of women's anxieties and demands for the procedure, not revised recommendations by the medical establishment.

concern over prescribing ERT for women with a history of breast cancer is that dormant tumor cells might be activated. There is surprisingly little clinical information to substantiate such concern."[15]

By then I was used to oncologists and epidemiologists finding "surprisingly little clinical information" to support the prohibition of HRT for breast cancer survivors. In 2000, Henk Verheul, a medical oncologist and now scientific co-director of the Cancer Center of Amsterdam, and his associates wrote that none of the current treatments for breast cancer—surgery, radiation, chemotherapy—were negatively affected by estrogen, even estrogens that were administered at concentrations that are *considerably higher* than those in typical prescriptions of HRT. The available studies, they concluded, "fail to demonstrate that, once breast cancer has been diagnosed, estrogens worsen prognosis, accelerate the course of the disease, reduce survival or interfere with the management of breast cancer. It may therefore be concluded that the prevalent opinion that estrogens and estrogen treatment are deleterious for breast cancer needs to be revisited."[16]

In Finland, Olavi Ylikorkala and Merja Metsä-Heikkilä, gynecological specialists and researchers at Helsinki University Central Hospital, observed that because the number of women surviving breast cancer has been increasing steadily, health professionals need to face the issue of how best to treat their symptoms of menopause and improve their health in general. (Ylikorkala's own research had documented the benefits of HRT in reducing the risk of vascular dementia and heart attacks in postmenopausal women.) The "categorical refusal [to prescribe HRT] is a double-edged sword because it also denies these women all the undisputable health benefits HRT provides," they said. "This refusal is not however supported by the observational data available so far on this question, because HRT has not increased the risk for breast cancer recurrence."[17]

Throughout the 1990s, wanting to make sure that my own study's findings were not an outlier, I kept track of any studies conducted anywhere in the world that compared breast cancer survivors given HRT with matched controls. None were the huge RCT trials of thousands of women that the FDA hoped someone would do someday. Some had small samples, some had larger ones; the length of time women were on HRT varied considerably; some followed up on their patients for a few months or two years or five years or longer. But take a look at the drumbeat of repeated findings that I read:

- Slovenia: Marjetka Uršič-Vrščaj and Sonja Bebar, at the Institute of Oncology in Ljubljana, compared twenty-one women with breast cancer who were treated with HRT for an average of twenty-eight months with two controls for each patient. They found no increased recurrence of breast cancer among the women on hormones.[18]

- Australia: John Eden, senior lecturer in reproductive endocrinology at the University of New South Wales, compared 90 breast cancer survivors treated with HRT for a median of eighteen months and followed for a median of seven years, with 180 matched controls. He found a small but significantly reduced recurrence of breast cancer among the women on hormones.[19]

- Australia: Jennifer Dew, a gynecologist at the Women's Health Institute of the Royal Hospital for Women, compared 167 women with a history of breast cancer who received HRT with 1,122 women with a similar history who were not given HRT. She found no increased recurrence of breast cancer among the women on hormones, even among women whose tumors were estrogen-receptor positive. Four years later, she updated her study with an even larger sample and again found that the use of HRT was not associated with an increased risk of recurrence of breast cancer.[20]

- Australia: Eva Durna, a gynecologist also at the University of New South Wales, reported a retrospective observational study of 286 breast cancer survivors given HRT compared with 686 breast cancer survivors who did not take HRT. (The women were followed for a median of under two years, but some had been on HRT for up to twenty-six years.) She found significantly lower rates of recurrence and rates of death from breast cancer in women who used HRT compared with nonusers. Two years later, she reported a second study of 524 women who were diagnosed with breast cancer when they were still premenopausal. Of the 277 who reached menopause following their diagnosis and treatment, 119 took HRT to control symptoms. The risks of recurrence of or death from breast cancer were no different among those women who took HRT and those who did not.[21]

- France: Marc Espie, an oncologist at the Hôpital Saint-Louis in Paris, followed 120 patients who received HRT after treatment for breast cancer, matching each patient with two comparable controls, for 2.4 years. He found no increased recurrence of breast cancer among the women on hormones.[22]

- Finland: Merja Marttunen and colleagues at University Central Hospital in Helsinki reported on 131 breast cancer survivors, 88 of whom had decided to use ERT and 43 of whom chose not to. All were followed for a mean of 2.6 years. The investigators found no increased recurrence of breast cancer among the women who chose estrogen.[23]
- Germany: Matthias Beckmann and colleagues at the Friedrich Alexander University in Erlangen retrospectively reviewed the records of 185 breast cancer patients, 64 of whom took HRT and 121 of whom did not. Even after five years, they found no increased recurrence of breast cancer among the women on hormones.[24]

Across the United States, researchers were coming to the same conclusion:

- Houston, Texas: Rena Vassilopoulou-Sellin, at the MD Anderson Cancer Center, conducted a randomized prospective study in which 39 breast cancer survivors were treated with Premarin and compared to 319 similar patients who did not receive hormones. After fifty-two months, she found no increased recurrence of breast cancer among the women on HRT.[25]
- Irvine, California: Wendy Brewster, a gynecologic oncologist and epidemiologist, and Philip DiSaia, director of the division of gynecologic oncology at the University of California, Irvine, matched 125 breast cancer patients who were taking ERT or HRT with 362 breast cancer patients who

received no hormones. They found no increased recurrence of breast cancer among the women on hormones.[26]

- Troy, Michigan: Medical oncologist David Decker reported a prospective study of 277 breast cancer survivors who received ERT for a mean duration of 3.7 years, matched with comparable controls. He found no increased recurrence of breast cancer among the women on hormones.[27]

- Dallas, Texas: George Peters, professor of surgery at the University of Texas Southwestern Medical Center, compared 64 breast cancer survivors treated with ERT after their diagnosis with 563 breast cancer survivors who received no ERT. After an average follow-up of twelve years, he found no increased recurrence of breast cancer among the women on hormones.[28]

- Seattle, Washington: Ellen O'Meara, a cancer researcher at the Fred Hutchinson Cancer Research Center of the University of Washington, reviewed the records of 2,755 women, ages thirty-five to seventy-four, who had been diagnosed with breast cancer between 1977 and 1999. Of those, 174 women were taking HRT after treatment. Each was matched with four control women identified from the same cohort over the same period and followed for a median of 3.7 years. "HRT after breast cancer has no adverse impact on recurrence and mortality," she concluded. Instead, she found significantly lower breast cancer recurrence rates, breast cancer mortality rates, and overall mortality rates among HRT users compared to nonusers.[29]

- Milwaukee, Wisconsin: In 2002, Linda N. Meurer and Sarah Lená, at the Medical College of Wisconsin, conducted a review of nine independent observational studies and one randomized controlled trial and found that breast cancer survivors using HRT had no increased risk of recurrence compared with controls. In their meta-analysis— totaling 717 women who used HRT after being diagnosed with breast cancer compared with 2,545 women who did not—they found that the survivors who were taking estrogen had significantly fewer deaths (3 percent) over the study periods than the women who were not (11.4 percent).[30]

Right now you are probably saying, "Wait! What about all the studies that found an increased risk of recurrence?" I thought you'd never ask. There weren't any. Until the Women's Health Initiative, this time with an ally: the HABITS study.

THE OPPOSITION WEIGHS IN

When the WHI published its findings in 2002, more than half of the six million women who had been taking HRT discontinued it within the year.[31] But three other events occurred almost immediately as well. First, research on hormones halted: of the eighteen reported studies that had begun in the 1990s in which survivors of breast and other cancers were being treated with HRT, virtually all of them stopped dead in their tracks. As far as I could determine, mine was the only one to continue recruiting patients and gathering data.

Second, the FDA added a black-box warning to the label of Prempro (Wyeth's version of HRT), and this caution remains today on all preparations of estrogen. It essentially states: "If you have ever had breast cancer, do not take this medication." The label also cautions that if the patient does take the hormones, she should take the smallest dose for the shortest time possible—an admonition no longer supported by evidence.

And third, thousands of lawsuits were filed almost immediately. A lawyer who represented Wyeth told me that at the height of litigation, Wyeth (and Pfizer, which had bought Wyeth) faced more than ten thousand lawsuits. About eight thousand cases in federal court were centralized in Arkansas, in a legal procedure that speeds the handling of complex liability suits. The others were spread out in state courts around the country. Of the dozens of trials, the results were mixed; the defense won some, and the plaintiffs won others. The largest plaintiffs' settlement was $78.74 million. "In a 2012 securities filing, Pfizer reported that it paid $896 million to resolve about 60% of the cases," the lawyer wrote. "The mass media, not good science, drove the litigation and the decisions of women with regard to their postmenopausal healthcare."[32]

Well, you say, of course an attorney representing Wyeth would complain that "the mass media, not good science, drove the litigation." But many oncologists, gynecologists, and researchers agree with that statement. "I have become somewhat frustrated since the WHI report," my colleague Phil DiSaia, at UC Irvine, wrote to me a few years later. "The media are not interested in facts. They seem to be focused on sensationalism. The fact that estrogen therapy alone carried no increase in the incidence of breast cancer was placed on page 18 in a small paragraph. Whereas, the borderline statistics on hormone replacement therapy was front-page news."[33]

DiSaia was especially disheartened by the paralyzing effect that the WHI had had on his own research. He had "become convinced that hormone replacement therapy is *not* contraindicated in breast cancer survivors and does *not* increase incidence of recurrence," and therefore he had been trying to launch a prospective, randomized study through the gynecologic oncology group at his medical school—the very study that the FDA had wanted done. "On each occasion the medical oncologists in the Group voted it down," he said, because of the WHI reports. At the time, they had nearly two thousand patients registered and ready for the study to begin.

The WHI was not the only punch. A second blow landed in 2004 with the publication of the HABITS study (an acronym formed from Hormonal Replacement Therapy After Breast Cancer—Is It Safe?). The WHI investigators immediately took the results to be a confirmation of their view that hormones were harmful in general and even more so for women who had had breast cancer. A leading WHI investigator, Rowan Chlebowski, wrote in an editorial about the HABITS study that it "may arguably not be the definitive word on the use of hormone therapy in women with breast cancer but it will probably be the last word when considered in context of our evolving understanding of the effects of hormone therapy on chronic disease in women."[34] Not the definitive word but the last word? What does that mean?

I read the HABITS report announcing the termination of the study with great interest. It appeared to contradict everything I've been telling you in this chapter, and it is still the most widely referenced study dealing with HRT for breast cancer survivors. The study, led by Lars Holmberg at the University Hospital's Regional Oncologic Center in Uppsala, Sweden, proposed to randomize 1,300 breast cancer survivors to HRT or no HRT and follow them for five years. The end point was the development of any new breast cancer—a recurrence in the original breast, a new lesion in the other breast, or a distant metastasis.

The study was prematurely terminated in 2003 after only two years of median follow-up and after only 434 women of the proposed 1,300 had been enrolled. The reason for the sudden termination was the disproportionate number of women on HRT who developed another breast cancer: twenty-six women in the HRT group (20 percent) and only seven in the non-HRT group (4 percent). Those numbers—twenty-six versus seven—seemed striking and important.[35] Few observers noticed that the groups did not differ in their incidence of metastatic disease or risk of death during that time, and when Premarin was used as the source of estrogen, there was no increased risk of breast cancer either.

The investigators updated their results in 2008 with follow-up on more participants.[36] The results were still concerning: this time, thirty-nine women in the HRT group (17.6 percent) and seventeen in the non-HRT group (7.7 percent) had developed new breast cancers. Again, however, there were some curious wrinkles: no new breast cancers among women who had had positive lymph-node involvement (which is believed to increase the risk of recurrence), no difference between groups in the incidence of distant metastases or in the risk of deaths from breast cancer, and no new breast cancers in women taking estrogen alone. And this time, the increased risk for women on HRT turned up only among those who were also taking tamoxifen. Now, this finding was most odd because it contradicted a host of research on tamoxifen in preventing recurrence of breast cancer, whether estrogen was taken with it or not, and it contradicted other studies that found no such increased risk for women taking both estrogen and tamoxifen.

Around the same time as the HABITS trial was being conducted, another study of HRT among Swedish breast cancer survivors, the Stockholm study, was under way. It was also a prospective randomized trial, similar in size to HABITS. Yet this study, in which 188 women were randomized to receive HRT and 190 got none, found no difference in the development of new breast cancers among HRT users as compared to nonusers, and like the HABITS trial, it found no difference in mortality between the two groups. At a ten-year follow-up, this finding was unchanged.[37]

Critics and professional societies weighed in on the HABITS study almost immediately. William Creasman, whose research in this area I previously described, noted some troubling problems: More than 20 percent of the women were not included in the analysis because they had not had at least one follow-up visit. The choice of hormone regimen — Premarin or other combinations of estrogen and progesterone — was left to the treating physician, so there was no uniformity in what was prescribed. Important risk factors in breast cancer are stage and status of lymph nodes, but this information was not provided at the time the women were randomized to get hormones or not. Why does this matter? You're a breast cancer survivor who has entered the study to see if hormones will increase or decrease your risk of recurrence. But the investigators don't give you a mammogram or conduct any other tests to see if you are currently cancer-free. Were the risk factors for recurrence the same in the two groups? We don't know.

Creasman seemed especially annoyed by the editorial commentary that accompanied the HABITS article. "This study can reasonably guide clinical practice of women with breast cancer," the editorial concluded. The hell it can, Creasman said, in essence, although he used the measured tones of medical writing: "This conclusion seems premature and without merit."[38]

When you have many studies pointing in one direction, and one renegade study that points the other way, you have to ask: What was wrong with all of the preceding studies, or why did this anomaly turn out as it did? Of the twenty studies published between 1980 and 2008, *only* the HABITS study found an increase in breast cancers among women on HRT, and *only* if they were also taking tamoxifen. Creasman wrote that he was unaware of any data that substantiated the belief in the harms of HRT for breast cancer survivors except for the HABITS study, which contained the flaws he'd enumerated. "With the exception of the HABITS study," he wrote, "all the other data do not identify the deleterious effects of replacement therapy in the post-cancer patient. To deny such therapy for life-disturbing symptoms does not seem to be in their best interest."[39] Alfred Mueck, head of the department of endocrinology and menopause at University Women's Hospital in Tübingen, Germany, and his colleagues agreed: a few prospective randomized studies and at least fifteen observational studies that investigated HRT after breast cancer were available, they wrote, and "only the [HABITS] study shows an increased risk of relapse."[40]

The Society of Obstetricians and Gynaecologists of Canada was not impressed by the HABITS study either. In 2005, its members issued a policy statement on the use of hormone replacement therapy after treatment of breast cancer that included these two summary points: "HRT after treatment of breast cancer has not been demonstrated to have an adverse impact on recurrence and mortality," and "HRT is an option in postmenopausal women with previously treated breast cancer."[41] But JoAnne Zujewski, head of Breast Cancer Therapeutics in the Clinical Investigation Branch at the National Cancer Institute, took the opposite view. "Combined with the negative results of the WHI, most U.S. physicians and their patients have gotten the message that long-term HRT can be harmful. The things they were trying to treat with hormone replacement therapy we now have better measures for," she said, "such as bisphosphonates for the prevention of osteoporosis and aspirin or statins for cardiac health."[42] This acceptance of faulty data for both the presumed harms of HRT and the allegedly equivalent benefits of its alternatives is, to my mind, reprehensible.

And so HABITS was not the definitive, or even the last, word after all. Far from providing a clear answer, it gave WHI supporters like Rowan Chlebowski and JoAnne Zujewski the chance to "see" the dangers of HRT, and it gave people like William Creasman, Phil DiSaia, and me the chance to "see" peculiar and improbable complications that muddied that conclusion. Even the HABITS study's lead investigator, Lars Holmberg, noted: "We agree that the results of a single randomized study should be interpreted cautiously, especially when the study is terminated early. We reported why we stopped recruitment in the HABITS trial and have not claimed to say 'the final word.'"[43]

Five years after the Women's Health Initiative study first appeared, I debated two of its supporters on a two-hour radio program in front of a studio audience, just after the pair had presented their data at the San Antonio Breast Cancer Symposium. Our debate was cordial, but it was clear to me that both men regarded my position with contempt.

"You'll find, Dr. Bluming," said one, an internationally respected biostatistician, "that statistics aren't everything."

"You should know," I replied. "You're the statistician."

During a break for station identification, he looked away from me and said loudly, so that everyone in the room could hear, "I believe that administering HRT to women with a history of breast cancer is malpractice." Remembering the surgeons who once thought it was malpractice to perform lumpectomies, all of the studies except HABITS that supported my position, and the gratitude of the many women in my own study, I could only offer to continue the debate.

Where are we today? While most new research stopped after the WHI, investigators have continued to reassess existing evidence with meta-analyses. Pelin Batur, an internist affiliated with the Cleveland Clinic, and her colleagues published a review of fifteen studies totaling 1,416 breast cancer survivors using hormone replacement therapy compared with a cumulative control group of 1,998 patients.[44] The majority of the women began HRT between two and five years after their diagnosis, and they remained on it for an average of three years. Compared to nonusers, the women on HRT had a 10 percent decreased chance of recurrence and even a slightly reduced mortality rate from cancer or other causes. Using the most recent data from the National Cancer Institute on rates of cancer incidence and survival in the United States, Batur calculated that the seven-year cancer-related mortality rate for invasive breast cancer was 17.9 percent for nonusers and 4.5 percent for the women on HRT.

THE TAKE-HOME

More than two decades ago, Melody Cobleigh and the Breast Cancer Committees of the Eastern Cooperative Oncology Group suggested a new guideline for the practice of medicine. "Clinical trials of ERT in breast cancer survivors have been hindered in part by the maxim *primum non nocere* (first do no harm)," they wrote. "Such moralizing prevents moral reflection. The task of moral reflection is to assess whether something is right or wrong. In light of the lack of evidence of a detrimental effect of ERT in breast cancer survivors and in light of the potential positive effects of ERT on the health of women, we suggest a new maxim, *primum certior fi, tunc mone* (first understand, then advise)."[45]

When my daughter was thirty-five, she discovered a tumor in her breast that turned out to be cancer. Because her mother, Martha, had been diagnosed at forty-seven, a fairly young age too, Martha underwent tests to see if she may have passed on a genetic predisposition to breast cancer. All the tests were negative. Our daughter had the tumor removed and received follow-up radiation. She had been unable to conceive even before the diagnosis, and eventually she had in vitro fertilization, which produced my granddaughter.

Twelve years later, when my daughter entered perimenopause, she asked me whether she should start HRT. We spoke at length and she read an early draft of this book. "Dad, I'm confused," she said. "Until now, whenever I needed advice on a medical course of action, you pointed me in the direction you felt was right. There was never any problem with your advice. So why won't you just tell me whether or not you think I should start HRT?"

I told my daughter what I would tell any reader of this book. "I cannot guarantee the cancer will not come back," I said, "with or without HRT. I want you to remain healthy through what I hope will be a long life to come, and I've provided you with the evidence of HRT's benefits and risks. Both you and I recognize that a decision not to take HRT has consequences—you would lose its many benefits—just as the decision to take it does."

I thought of the wise observation of Siddhartha Mukherjee: "It's easy to make perfect decisions with perfect information," he wrote in *The Laws of Medicine*. "Medicine asks you to make perfect decisions with imperfect information."[46]

On my advice, but with her full understanding, my daughter decided to take HRT.

7

Progesterone and the Pill

Over the years, when Avrum has written or lectured about the benefits of HRT and misconceptions about the harms of estrogen, he is often asked what he calls the "what-about" questions:

What about progesterone? "I know for me, personally," one woman wrote to Av in an e-mail, "the dilemma is no longer about taking estrogen, but rather about what to do concerning progesterone, which seems to have become the new villain. I've even contemplated having my uterus removed so as not to have to take progesterone and not subject myself to all its downsides, although that feels ridiculously radical to me." (It is.)

What about birth control pills? "My daughter is on the pill," wrote an older woman, "but I remember the early days when the pill had very high estrogen levels and I've been suspicious about it ever since. Should I worry? Does the pill increase her risk of breast cancer?"

Let's look at the evidence.

What About Progesterone?

Progesterone was isolated and purified in the early 1930s by scientists in several countries who together agreed to call it *progesterone* because it is the hormone that supports pregnancy (pro-gestation). Progesterone stimulates the cells in the uterine lining to proliferate in preparation for the possible arrival of a fertilized egg. The level of circulating progesterone increases during the latter half of the menstrual cycle but declines back to its resting level if fertilization does not occur. If it does, the level of progesterone continues to rise, stimulating the endometrial cells to provide a nourishing environment for the fetus.

Today, the word *progesterone* is often misleadingly applied to a variety of related but different preparations. In the United States, the most commonly used natural form of this hormone is micronized progesterone, sold as Prometrium. In contrast, *progestins* are synthetic compounds that mimic the activity of progesterone. The most frequently prescribed progestin in this country is medroxyprogesterone acetate (MPA, sold as Provera). Prempro, a common form of hormone replacement therapy, is a combination of estrogen and MPA; this was the kind of HRT used in the Women's Health Initiative study.

We can answer Av's first questioner right off the bat: keep your uterus and take the progesterone. But she was right to observe that progesterone "seems to have become the new villain." The WHI's study in 2002 reported that estrogen on its own did not increase the risk of breast cancer; in fact, as we've discussed, over the ensuing years in which they did follow-ups, it was associated with a decreased risk.[1] As one researcher summarized: "The only statistically significant outcome for all participants (50–79 years) in the WHI Estrogen-Alone Trial for the 13-year cumulative long-term follow-up was a reduction in invasive breast cancer with CEE [Premarin]."[2]

And so, to continue making the case against HRT, the WHI investigators and their supporters began to argue that it was the addition of progesterone that was harmful.[3] Many more women take HRT than ERT, and those women understandably became worried. Once again, however, considerable evidence exonerates progesterone. In fact, as with estrogen, it is often used as a treatment:

- In 1986, Hendrik Van Veelen and his colleagues in the department of medicine at Deaconess Hospital, Leeuwarden, the Netherlands, conducted a prospective, randomized study of postmenopausal patients with advanced breast cancer. Half were treated with the progestin MPA and half with tamoxifen. They found that 44 percent of those treated with progestin had a partial or complete remission, compared to 35 percent of the women treated with tamoxifen. In fact, MPA was even more effective than tamoxifen in the treatment of bone metastases and in the treatment of women over seventy. A 1993 review of all published randomized clinical trials comparing tamoxifen with progestins for metastatic breast cancer in postmenopausal women confirmed these findings.[4]

- In a randomized controlled trial of one thousand women about to have surgery for breast cancer, Rajendra Badwe, a surgical oncologist in Mumbai, India, injected half of them with a single dose of progesterone five to fourteen days before operating. Five years later, this injection had significantly improved the disease-free prognosis for women who had positive node involvement compared to those who did not receive the progesterone.[5] (The women with no lymph-node involvement already had a favorable prognosis.)

- Women who have a progesterone deficiency—for example, because they suffer from a chronic condition in which they fail to ovulate—have a higher risk of developing breast cancer; in one controlled study of more than a thousand premenopausal women with progesterone deficiency, the risk was five times as high.[6]

- Epidemiologist Brian Strom (now retired) and colleagues at the Center for Clinical Epidemiology and Biostatistics at the University of Pennsylvania conducted a study of 4,575 randomly selected women, ages thirty-five to sixty-four, who had survived invasive breast cancer. Comparing these women with 4,682 controls, they found that taking progestin-only contraceptives for four years did not increase the risk of recurrence of the cancer.[7]

Progesterone may improve breast cancer survival rates. In 2015, Hisham Mohammed and his team at the University of Adelaide's Dame Roma Mitchell Cancer Research Laboratories reported that receptors that mediate the activity of estrogen and progesterone interact with DNA to control the growth of a large majority of breast cancers. Their discovery may bode well for targeted treatments. Two years later, Jason Carroll, at the University of Cambridge's Cancer Research UK Institute, reported that natural progesterone can stimulate the progesterone receptor on a breast cancer cell, resulting in suppression of its growth.[8]

Well, then, some investigators suggested, perhaps it's not the natural, purer forms of progesterone that are the problem so much as progestins, the synthetic versions that were used in the Women's Health Initiative. Guess who promoted that idea? Right. The data linking the combination of estrogen and progestin to an increased risk of breast cancer came largely from the WHI, whose own findings on this matter, as we have seen, were barely statistically significant and inconsistent across their follow-up reports. Indeed, some investigators have argued that the WHI did not find a true increased risk but a statistically spurious one.[9] Even if that increased risk were worth writing home about, it should be put in perspective, which Richard Santen, an endocrinologist and professor of medicine at the University of Virginia, and his colleagues thoughtfully did. They themselves do not think HRT should be taken for more than a few years because of its presumed risks of breast cancer, but they acknowledged that the risk is low. "Based on the worst-case analysis," they wrote, "a 50-year-old woman taking an estrogen/progestin combination of HRT for 10 [years] has only a 4% chance of getting breast cancer. Without HRT, the risk would be 2%. These statistics sound more reassuring if expressed as the number of women remaining free of breast cancer. For example, women taking HRT for 10 [years] have a 96% chance of remaining free of breast cancer vs. 98% of those not taking HRT."[10]

It is still not known why progestins should have a slightly higher risk than progesterone. Some progestins stimulate androgen receptors (which both women and men have, though obviously in different proportions), and high levels of free testosterone (an androgen) have been identified as a risk factor in breast cancer both before and after menopause.[11] An animal study that supports some concern about progestins was conducted by the obstetrician-gynecologist Angiolo Gadducci and his team at the University of Pisa. They removed the ovaries of adult female monkeys and then randomly assigned them to be given estrogen plus progestin or a placebo. The monkeys on the progestin developed a greater proliferation of the single layer of epithelial cells that line the breast's milk ducts. When the monkeys were put on micronized (natural) progesterone instead of progestin, no increased proliferation of cells occurred.[12] Again, the precise biological mechanism behind this result is unclear, but perhaps one reason is that micronized progesterone does not stimulate androgen receptors as progestins do. In 2005, an extensive literature review by another obstetrician-gynecologist, Carlo Campagnoli, and his colleagues at the Sant'Anna Gynecological Hospital in Turin, Italy, concluded that using oral micronized progesterone eliminated any increased risk of breast cancer associated with HRT.[13]

Don't throw out your Provera just yet! It might seem from these studies that women who wish to be on HRT should, to feel safest, take progesterone in its oral, micronized form. Yet even so, we are talking about extremely small differences in risks between progesterone and progestin—no more than a 2 percent bump. Some women, including Av's wife, Martha, do better in terms of side effects with Provera (the progestin) than with micronized progesterone, and they should not be unduly concerned. And remember that even if HRT with progestin increases the risk of breast cancer by 2 percent, we have bombarded you with evidence that women on HRT live longer and have a lower death rate from breast cancer than those not taking HRT.

There's one other important consideration to keep in mind about the benefits of HRT: it appreciably reduces the risk of colon cancer, the third most common cancer in the United States. In 2018, the projections were nearly one hundred thousand new cases every year and a much too high 52 percent mortality rate.[14] However, the rate of developing colon cancer is consistently lower for women, especially premenopausal women, suggesting that estrogen protects against the growth of cancerous cells in the colon.[15] Over the decades, numerous researchers have found that women who take HRT in pill form (as opposed to the transdermal patch) have a lower risk of getting colon cancer and a lower mortality rate from colon cancer if they do get it as compared with women not on hormones.[16] Not all studies have gotten these results,[17] but the preponderance of them have. Even the Women's Health Initiative did. In an analysis of all women enrolled in the WHI, cancer researcher Arthur Hartz at the Huntsman Cancer Institute of the University of Utah and his colleagues found that the use of any form of HRT reduces the risk of colon cancer by 30 percent. A similar study found that both estrogen alone and estrogen plus progestin—administered in any form, patch or pill—were associated with a "strong reduction" in the risk of colon cancer.[18]

WHAT ABOUT BIRTH CONTROL PILLS?

The first oral contraceptive, Enovid, was approved in 1960, although it was illegal for unmarried women to use it (or any other birth control, for that matter) in twenty-six states. Five years later, in its landmark decision *Griswold v. Connecticut*, the Supreme Court ruled that it was unconstitutional for the government to prohibit married couples from using birth control. The court did not quite get up the nerve to legalize birth control for all American women until 1972, in *Eisenstadt v. Baird*.

The estrogen most commonly used in birth control pills is ethinyl estradiol. In the early years, when the pill contained relatively high doses of estrogen (Enovid had as much as 10 milligrams of ethinyl estradiol), a small but worrying number of women developed blood clots in their veins, usually in the legs. Sometimes, fragments of those clots broke off and traveled to the lungs, leading to pulmonary emboli and, in some cases, death.[19] This lethal complication was clearly unacceptable, and the shock of its occurring in otherwise healthy young women caused a national uproar. As a result, the dose of hormones in these pills was cut way down, and emboli are now extremely rare.[20] In today's oral contraceptives, ethinyl estradiol comes in a variety of dosages. Some are higher than the dose used in HRT, and some are lower. Some low-dose oral contraceptives contain only 0.01 milligram of ethinyl estradiol and tend to be prescribed primarily for perimenopausal women who want contraception but who also have irregular or heavy menses or hormonally related symptoms that impair quality of life. These preparations provide adequate estrogen to relieve hot flashes and other vasomotor symptoms.[21] (The progesterone components of birth control pills and HRT are often similar.)

At any of these doses, oral contraceptives are among the most effective birth control methods we have, with failure rates of less than 1 percent when used as directed. We also now have nearly sixty years of research on their safety, and for women who are concerned about estrogen and breast cancer, the findings are immensely reassuring—even for breast cancer survivors:

- Throughout the 1980s, a series of large-scale studies from the Centers for Disease Control's Cancer and Steroid Hormone (CASH) Study repeatedly found no significant association between oral contraceptive use and breast cancer, even when it was used at an early age, before first pregnancy, at the time of diagnosis, or in women with a family history of breast cancer.[22]
- In 2002, another report from the CDC evaluated 4,574 women with breast cancer and 4,682 controls. More than 75 percent of these women were using or had used oral contraceptives. The researchers found no increased risk of breast cancer associated with duration of oral contraceptive use or age at which a woman began taking it (including those younger than twenty).[23]
- In 2007, a large British cohort study of 46,000 women, half of whom took oral contraceptives and all of whom had been followed for an average of twenty-four years, found no difference in breast cancer incidence among oral contraceptive users compared to never-users.[24]
- In 2008, Jane Figueiredo, an epidemiologist and professor of preventive medicine at USC's Keck School of Medicine, and her colleagues conducted the WECARE study (for Women's Environment, Cancer, and Radiation Epidemiology), a population-based, case-control study of 708 women who had had cancer in both breasts and 1,395 women who had had cancer in one breast. They found that oral contraceptive

use either before or after the development of primary breast cancer did not increase the risk of cancer developing in the opposite breast. The risk did not increase with longer duration of use or among women who began taking birth control pills at a younger age. Two years later, in a follow-up study of women with primary breast cancer who were also BRCA1 or BRCA2 mutation carriers, they again found no association between use of oral contraceptives and risk of breast cancer developing in the opposite breast.[25]

- In 2010, the Nurses' Health Study reported that among 1,344 breast cancer patients, a very few (only 57, to be precise) who had been on birth control pills for more than eight years had a small increased risk of breast cancer, and this small increased risk was seen only among those who were taking a progestin known to stimulate androgen receptors. Because of the very low numbers of these patients, however, the authors concluded that "current oral contraceptive use is not a major cause of breast cancer."[26]

- In 2013, a meta-analysis of thirteen prospective studies involving 11,722 cases of breast cancer among 850,000 women found no significant association between the use of oral contraceptives (past or present) and breast cancer.[27]

- As with other findings about estrogen, survival rates for breast cancer patients tend to be higher in women taking oral contraceptives at the time of their diagnosis than in women not taking estrogen.[28]

But here is some truly stunning news. The number of ovarian cancers diagnosed in the United States each year is about 10 percent of the number of newly diagnosed breast cancers—22,000 ovarian cancers compared to 220,000 breast cancers. Ovarian cancer is much more difficult to treat and cure; there's still no good screening test for it; and, in 2018, its mortality rate (63 percent) remained many times higher than that of newly diagnosed breast cancer.[29] Yet the available evidence suggests that oral contraceptives decrease the risk of ovarian cancer by 40 to 80 percent.[30] In one study, epidemiologist Martin Vessey and his colleague Rosemary Painter, in the department of public health at the University of Oxford, looked at more than 17,000 women recruited from family-planning clinics between 1968 and 1974 and followed until 2004. Women who had been taking oral contraceptives were 40 percent less likely to develop ovarian cancer than women who had never taken the pill. Moreover, women taking the pill for more than ten years reduced their overall risk of ovarian cancer by as much as 80 percent, and this benefit persisted for nearly twenty years after they stopped oral contraception.[31]

As we said in chapter 1, when you are dealing with epidemiological studies, whether of small or large populations, you will never get 100 percent concordance in results. That's why we must look for the picture that emerges from the larger mosaic formed by all the pieces of evidence, even if a few don't fit. With the question of birth control pills and breast cancer, as usual, a few pieces don't fit, and those pieces—showing a small but significant increase in the risk of breast cancer among women taking oral contraceptives— should be noted.

In 1996, the Collaborative Group on Hormonal Factors in Breast Cancer performed a meta-analysis of fifty-four epidemiologic studies from around the world on oral contraceptive use and invasive breast cancer.[32] After reanalyzing data from 53,297 women with breast cancer and 100,239 women without breast cancer, they found that women taking oral contraceptives had a small increased risk of developing invasive breast cancer, a risk that remained for ten years after stopping the pill. It was, however, a very small increased risk. How small? Small enough that when a subsequent review was published in 2004, the authors waved it away. Because rates of breast cancer among women young enough to be on birth control were so low, they said this time, and because the absolute numbers of women in the sample who developed breast cancer were, accordingly, very small, any apparent increase in breast cancer risk due to birth control pills was trivial.[33]

Nevertheless, as night follows day and penguins follow fish, scare stories will ever be upon us. They are...scary. They get our attention. They draw readers. They sell. And so, predictably, in 2017, a friend called us to ask about a *New York Times* article that worried her:

Birth Control Pills Still Linked to Breast Cancer, Study Finds

The headline was dramatic, as was the subhead: "Women Using Birth Control Pills and I.U.D.s That Release Hormones Face a Higher Risk Than Those Using Methods Without Hormones, Scientists in Denmark Reported."[34] The story described an article that had just been published in the *New England Journal of Medicine,* a prospective nationwide cohort study involving 1.8 million Danish women between the ages of fifteen and forty-nine who had been followed for ten years. The researchers found an increase in breast cancers among current and recent users of oral contraceptives and in women using IUDs that released progestin.[35]

The *New York Times* reporter, Roni Caryn Rabin, noted right away that the "absolute risk was small." In fact, in an accompanying editorial in the *NEJM* titled "Oral Contraceptives and the Small Increased Risk of Breast Cancer," David J. Hunter, a professor of epidemiology and medicine at the University of Oxford, emphasized how small it was: "An increase of around one new breast cancer case per 7,690 current and recent users of hormonal contraception." He placed the findings in the context of previous research, including the studies that found an increased risk, such as the one from the Collaborative Group on Hormonal Factors in Breast Cancer, and those that did not, such as the Centers for Disease Control reports. He concluded, as the Collaborative Group had, that the clinical implications of this study "must be placed in the context of the low incidence rates of breast cancer among younger women," pointing out that most of the new breast cancer cases occurring in the study were among women over the age of forty who were still on the pill. Most important, he wrote, "the risk of breast cancer needs to be balanced against the benefits of the use of oral contraceptives," and the risks were far outweighed by the pill's many impressive benefits: it provided effective contraception, helped women who have painful menstrual periods or abnormally heavy bleeding, and was associated with substantial reductions in the risks of ovarian, endometrial, and colorectal cancers later in life.[36]

As if to underscore the point, the reporter inserted this link smack in the middle of her story:

[ALSO READ: Birth Control Pills Protect Against Cancer, Too]

Indeed they do, as a 2018 study in the *Journal of the American Medical Association: Oncology* reported. Kara Michels and her associates at the Division of Cancer Epidemiology and Genetics of the National Cancer Institute published the results of a prospective analysis of more than 196,536 women, followed from 1995 to 2011. Approximately half of the women were taking oral contraceptives at the time they enrolled in the study. The researchers found a 40 percent reduction in the incidence of ovarian cancer in the women who had been taking oral contraceptives for at least ten years, and a similar reduction in the incidence of endometrial cancer. They found no association between oral contraception and the likelihood of developing breast cancer.[37]

The Take-Home

Because many women are concerned about the possible risks of progesterone and birth control pills, let's review:

- The word *progesterone,* the natural hormone that supports pregnancy (pro-gestation), is often applied to different preparations. The most commonly used natural form is micronized progesterone (Prometrium). In contrast, progestins are synthetic compounds that mimic the activity of progesterone. In the United States, the most frequently prescribed progestin is medroxyprogesterone acetate (MPA, sold as Provera).
- Although progesterone seems to have become a "new villain" in arguments against HRT, the preponderance of evi-

dence exonerates it. As with estrogen, progesterone is often used as an effective treatment for women with breast cancer and may even improve breast cancer survival rates.

- Investigators have reported no increased risk of breast cancer among women on HRT when the form of progesterone was oral (natural) micronized progesterone; they found a very small increase in risk—only 2 percent—when the progesterone was a synthetic progestin. Nonetheless, some women who take HRT do better with a progestin than with micronized progesterone. They should not be concerned because of the more important overall finding that women on HRT live longer and have a significantly lower death rate from breast cancer than those not taking HRT.

- Women on ERT or any formulation of HRT have a significant reduction in the risk of colon cancer.

- Oral contraceptives are overwhelmingly safe and highly effective. Most studies, such as those from the Centers for Disease Control, have repeatedly found no association between use of oral contraceptives and breast cancer. This finding holds regardless of how young a woman was when she began taking the pill, whether she used it before her first pregnancy, whether she was on the pill at the time of diagnosis, and whether she has a family history of breast cancer.

The challenge, researchers and physicians agree, is to neither ignore small risks nor inflate them into looming dangers. "Nothing is risk-free, and hormonal contraceptives are not an exception to that rule," Øjvind Lidegaard, one of the study's authors, told the *New York Times*. As we have stressed repeatedly, every medical intervention, whether it is a diagnostic test, surgery, or medication, carries a risk. Even something that might seem to be entirely beneficial, such as vitamins, can have risks when misused or overused; for example, cases of hypervitaminosis A and hypervitaminosis D, potentially lethal conditions resulting from overdoses of A and D, respectively, have been reported. Conversely, most people who watch pharmaceutical ads on TV now tune out the obligatory warnings, a list that includes everything from rashes to death. The list is usually so long that it becomes comical (hence the parodies that the drug being advertised could grow hair on your elbows or cause a foot to fall off).

But the counter-problem of people ignoring serious warnings is their taking trivial warnings too seriously. As we noted in the previous chapter, in the wake of the Women's Health Initiative reports, the FDA stipulated that all hormone therapy products, including vaginal creams with estrogen, must have boxed warnings to alert users to the "risks" of heart attacks, strokes, blood clots, breast cancer, and dementia. In a 2017 editorial for *Menopause: The Journal of the North American Menopause Society,* Cynthia Stuenkel wrote, "Many clinicians have experienced the dismay of prescribing vaginal estrogen, only to have their patient return in follow-up with the news that after reading the patient package insert, she (or her partner) had decided not to chance the perils as highlighted in the boxed warning."[38] No wonder. Comfortable sex probably isn't worth a stroke, cancer, or dementia!

But wonders never cease, and progress marches on. In January 2018, the Women's Health Initiative investigators announced that the dose of estrogen in vaginal creams is not associated with an increased risk of breast cancer.[39] It took them only sixteen years, so who knows—maybe in another sixteen years, they will change their minds about HRT too.

8

Debates, Decisions, and Final
Lessons in the Case for HRT

In this final chapter, Avrum will describe the challenge of trying to find common ground with colleagues who disagree with
him, review the benefits and risks of HRT, and answer some
key questions that his patients ask him—questions, we imagine,
that you may have also. For readers of this book whose physicians
still closely adhere to guidelines informed by the Women's Health
Initiative, Av has provided a list of its ten key problems in hopes
that it may prove a useful start for conversation.

*   *   *

Many years ago, I was invited to debate Susan Love, then the director of the UCLA Breast Center, on the topic of estrogen and breast
cancer for an audience of physicians and cancer researchers in
Southern California. As the guest speaker, I was first. I started by

saying I felt sure that everyone, including Susan, would leave the debate having reached some point of agreement, because, after all, we had the same goal: the prevention and eradication of breast cancer. I presented my case, summarizing the gist of what you have read in this book, and then I sat down to hear her response to the evidence and conclusions I had offered.

Love began by saying she would never agree with me because she objected strongly to the idea that menopause was a disease, and anyone who suggested that hormone replacement therapy had any benefits was clearly labeling menopause a disease that needed treatment. Girls did very well until they reached the age of puberty, she said, and then they spent the next several decades on a tumultuous emotional and physical roller coaster. Only after menopause, she said, do we get women like Eleanor Roosevelt, Indira Gandhi, Golda Meir, and the many postmenopausal suffragists who helped women get the right to vote. (She overlooked the fact that all of these women had been activists all their lives.) The problem, Love concluded, wasn't that women suffered estrogen deficiency following menopause; it was that they suffered "estrogen poisoning" between puberty and menopause.

Her remarks were followed by dead silence.

Susan Love went on to become director of what is now the Dr. Susan Love Research Foundation and write popular books. Among them is *Dr. Susan Love's Menopause and Hormone Book: Making Informed Choices,* which repeats the estrogen-poisoning line and lists the other benefits of menopause, a time, she says, when women no longer feel "constrained by the dictates of finding a man for reproduction."[1] She continues to promote the view that the "medicalization" of menopause is bad for women, an unnecessary intrusion into a completely normal aspect of women's lives.

Still, it was easier for me to debate Susan Love, whose position was clear, if simplistic, than to debate, on separate occasions over the ensuing years, the eminent physicians and epidemiologists who either worked with the WHI, supported its primary claims, or were convinced that estrogen was a carcinogen. One such expert is Malcolm Pike, who has a PhD in mathematical statistics and is a former director of the Cancer Epidemiology Unit at Oxford University, a former director of the USC epidemiology department, and now an attending epidemiologist at Memorial Sloan Kettering Cancer Center, where he is identified as "a renowned epidemiologist who has made seminal contributions to the understanding of hormone-related breast cancer." Pike's position has long been that breast cancer *is* related to hormone levels, and by now you know why I believe that position, no matter how many prominent experts hold it, is unsupported by a vast number of disconfirming studies.

During my debate with Pike in 2003, in front of an audience of physicians attending a continuing medical education program, I sought common ground, as I always try to do. "We agree," I said to him, "that the incidence of breast cancer continues to rise through and past menopause, even in women who are not on HRT. If estrogen were really a cause of breast cancer, shouldn't that rate decline — indeed, shouldn't it drop precipitously, given that levels of circulating estrogen drop so sharply following menopause?" He agreed that rates of breast cancer continue to rise in older women as their estrogen levels fall. But, he countered, the *rate of increase* slows as estrogen drops.

I thought, *Pardon me?* Aloud I asked, "How does this bear on my argument? The point is that rates of breast cancer continue to rise steadily into old age. If estrogen is a primary contributor to breast cancer, those rates should steadily decline. Why don't they?"

"I'm not a real doctor the way Dr. Bluming is," Pike joked to the audience. "All I have is a PhD, not an MD, but my PhD is in statistics" — the implication being that his possession of that degree was an adequate answer.

In 2007, I had the opportunity to debate Peter Ravdin, MD, PhD, on a radio show during the San Antonio Breast Cancer Symposium; we discussed the relation of HRT to breast cancer. Ravdin, director of the Breast Health Clinic at the University of Texas, later won a Pathfinder Award from the American Society of Breast Disease, celebrating him as "an innovator who has combined biological intuition, clinical and translational research, and clinical practice with an interdisciplinary understanding to advance the fight against breast disease and breast cancer." During our debate, Ravdin noted that the incidence of breast cancer declined within eight months after the first report of the Women's Health Initiative in 2002, and, for want of an alternative explanation, he attributed that decline to the fact that the number of HRT prescriptions had nose-dived and women were no longer taking that risky estrogen-progestin combination.

"Unfortunately for that argument," I countered, "that decline started in 1999, long before the 2002 publication of the WHI. Moreover, most breast cancers take a long time to become diagnosable tumors — far longer than eight months."

Well, Ravdin said, actually he was talking about the very small, not-yet-diagnosed, "subclinical" cancers of the breast that, he conjectured, stopped growing when HRT was discontinued.[2]

"That might be a credible position," I replied, "if the decreased incidence we see in the national rates were due primarily to a decrease in those small or even noninvasive breast cancers you are describing. But it isn't; the primary decrease is occurring in larger, invasive tumors, which take far longer to develop than eight months. Besides, there has been no decline in breast cancer rates among black women. Besides, the overwhelming majority of women who take HRT do not develop breast cancer, and the overwhelming majority of women who do develop breast cancer do not take HRT—and you have no evidence that the decline occurred *only* among women who had been on HRT and stopped. And by the way, in Norway, where women went off HRT following the Women's Health Initiative at the same rates as here, there was no decline in breast cancer. How, then, can you claim credit on behalf of the WHI for a decline in breast cancer rates in America but not Norway, and only among white women?"

He had no reply except to repeat his conviction that the WHI had saved many lives by getting women off HRT. That year, in a published exchange in *JAMA* in which I and several other writers criticized the WHI for taking credit for the decline in breast cancer rates, Ravdin and his colleagues still maintained that "although there is no conclusive proof of a causal link between coincident sharp declines in the use of hormone-replacement therapy and the incidence of estrogen-receptor-positive breast cancer, we have yet to see a credible alternative explanation."[3] What does that mean? It means we can't explain the decline in breast cancer rates, but we'll cheerfully take credit for it.

Malcolm Pike and Peter Ravdin are giants in their fields, deservedly honored. But their eminence should not blind us to the inherent contradiction in their arguments. Ravdin says that when estrogen declines because women go off HRT, breast cancer declines. Pike says that when estrogen declines as women age, breast cancer rates rise—but "at a slower rate," whatever that means. Both of these men are twisting the evidence to fit their preconceived beliefs.

I have been reading comments by the WHI investigators for many years. Some individuals among them have dogmatically stuck to their original positions, still maintaining that the WHI was *the* very best study ever and therefore has the most reliable conclusion about HRT—namely, that HRT causes breast cancer. Others have cautiously admitted that maybe all those early scare stories were, well, premature and a bit overblown. In 2007, only five years after those "Stop the presses! HRT causes breast cancer and deaths from other diseases too!" press releases and headlines, a writer for *Scientific American* asked several leaders of the Women's Health Initiative for their current views.[4]

"With hindsight you could say, well, maybe we should have emphasized reasonable use even more," said Jacques Rossouw, the cardiologist who headed the project and who, as noted in chapter 1, had wanted for years *before* the WHI to slow down the HRT "bandwagon."

Discussing the abrupt termination of the WHI, Marcia Stefanick said, "Maybe we didn't need to do it that way. It wasn't an emergency—it wasn't like people were, you know, under serious threat of the adverse outcomes." She waited five years to say this? The entire thrust of the WHI's first announcement was that there *was* a "serious threat" to women of adverse outcomes. Stefanick added, "I wish we had figured out a way to change prescribing practices but have fewer people distressed about it." I can think of a few ways: Don't rush to press without your entire team having read and agreed on your *JAMA* article; consider measured ways of presenting your data; and, by the way, make sure your data are solid.

And JoAnn Manson offered her thoughts: "Taking all of the previous research into account, there may have been a reason to look very closely at differences by age and differences by time since menopause.... Had that been part of the earliest reports, it might have helped put the results into perspective for younger women." There "may" have been a reason? There certainly was.

Other investigators have conducted subsequent reanalyses that contradicted their earlier conclusions, but instead of acknowledging error, they typically waffle, unable to say a good word for HRT even when their own evidence shows that they can. For example, in a 2012 article published in *Lancet Oncology,* the WHI investigators were already backtracking on their claims about estrogen and breast cancer. Women on estrogen alone, they reported, were less likely to die of breast cancer—indeed, less likely to die from all causes after a breast cancer diagnosis—than women assigned to placebo.[5] Yet the report's lead author, Garnet Anderson, told the *Seattle Times* that "the results were not favorable for women with a family history of breast cancer" (untrue, as we saw in chapter 1, where we discussed the research on BRCA-positive women); that the "combination-pill trial, closed in 2002, found women taking Prempro...had a higher risk of breast cancer" (untrue; the risk was not statistically significant); that "the estrogen-only trial, shut down in 2004, found a risk of stroke and no protection from heart attacks" (not accurate, as we saw in chapter 3); and that "we can't say what would happen if these women stayed on estrogen for 10 or 15 years" (yes, we can; we have ample data from the many studies of women who have taken hormones for ten, fifteen, and twenty years).[6]

What about their important finding of fewer deaths among women on estrogen? Anderson advised caution because "the mortality data are thin." But those findings were statistically significant, and plenty of other studies support the conclusion that HRT prolongs women's lives. Yet she was satisfied enough with "thin data" when she and her fellow investigators could fatten them up to worry the public with nonsignificant claims that HRT increases the risk of death from all causes. She chose caution only when dealing with good news. On one of the most important findings from her own project—that when taken during the "window of benefit" after the onset of menopause, HRT confers protection against heart attacks and strokes—Anderson was silent. By the way, she is not a physician; she is a biostatistician.

Or consider JoAnn Manson's assessment in 2015, in which she wrote that while she still believed that HRT increased the risk of breast cancer, she was willing to agree that the risk was "offset" by the protection HRT affords against bone fractures, diabetes, and endometrial cancer. Seemingly having forgotten the WHI's early claim that HRT increases rates of "all-cause mortality," she said that it all balances out. "We can reassure women now," she told the *Times* (UK). "Even though there are risks, there are counterbalancing benefits that mean the effect on mortality is neutral."[7] That is something of an understatement—contradicted by the WHI's own evidence. In a continuing analysis published in *JAMA* in 2017, Manson and her colleagues reported that women who had taken ERT or HRT and been followed for up to eighteen years had *no* extra deaths from heart disease, breast cancer, any other kind of cancer, or, for that matter, from any other disease compared to the control group of women who were not taking hormones.[8]

Where were the press releases and headlines saying "Sorry, everyone, that we scared you; we overreacted"?

When Carol and I talk with friends about the arguments in this book, they often respond with something to the effect of "What the hell? Why did the WHI investigators proceed as they did? Why did they raise frightening alarms when none were warranted? What were their motives?" And we always reply that we doubt that the investigators had nefarious goals or an intent to deceive. Rather, it seems likely that they were simply so convinced that estrogen and HRT were harmful that they massaged their data to confirm that hypothesis. You may recall the words in chapter 1 of a senior WHI investigator who responded to a question about why the WHI had inflated the importance of breast cancer risks that were not statistically significant: if it's an important question and you can't do the study again because it costs too much money, he said, "the statistical police have to leave the room." And then there was Rossouw, eager to stop that bandwagon.

Steven Sloman and Philip Fernbach, in *The Knowledge Illusion: Why We Never Think Alone,* noted that "scientific attitudes are not based on rational evaluation of evidence, and therefore providing information does not change them. Attitudes are determined instead by a host of contextual and cultural factors that make them largely immune to change."[9] As we surveyed the many decades of research and debate about menopausal hormones, that is precisely what we found. Over the past seventy years, the evidence of HRT's benefits and risks—evidence converging from animal studies, human studies, observational studies, randomized controlled studies, pilot studies, and clinical studies—has pretty much remained the same. But the interpretations of that evidence have changed according to the "contextual and cultural factors" that, at any given time in our society, have shaped whether women and their physicians think that hormone "replacement" is good or bad, healthy or detrimental, feminist or antifeminist.

A different response to our argument has come from those physicians, epidemiologists, and women's health activists we have written to, people whose opinions we deeply value and whom we hold in great regard, who believe that the WHI was a valuable and groundbreaking study. At their express invitations, we sent them our published articles in the *Cancer Journal* and *Climacteric* and said, "Please tell us where we are wrong. Look where we reanalyzed the WHI's own conclusions; did we go off the rails somewhere? Look at all that data mining they did to squeak out significant results. Look at how unrepresentative in age and health their sample was, yet they freely extrapolated their findings to all menopausal women. Is what they did okay with you?" Two colleagues replied, in essence, that the Women's Health Initiative was a randomized controlled study, and that's all they needed to know; whatever its flaws, it was the best research we have to date and would likely ever have. Others, taking Susan Love's position, said, in essence, "You will never persuade me that taking hormones can be beneficial for women." Most of our correspondents, however, did not respond.

We understand that silence. It's a pain in the neck to explain to someone why you are committed to a hypothesis (for example, that HRT causes cancer or that the medicalization of menopause is bad for women) when you regard that hypothesis as being as obvious and universally accepted as the fact that the earth is round. If one of the loonies who endorse the flat-earth view—incredibly, they have been proliferating in conspiracy corners of the internet— asked us to justify our position that the earth is round, we wouldn't reply, and you probably wouldn't either. Of course, serious scientists endeavor to address differences of opinion, interpretations of data, and basic hypotheses during the process of peer review and arguments in professional journals. But the more committed they are to the truths they hold to be self-evident, the less motivated they are to entertain an opponent's position. It's much easier to ignore that person's position than engage in an argument about it.

Those who defend the WHI make many claims to support their view about estrogen's harms—for example, that increased lifetime exposure to hormones (early menarche and late menopause) increases the risk of breast cancer, or that tamoxifen works as an anti-estrogen, so therefore its effectiveness is evidence of estrogen's carcinogenic quality. In chapter 1, we gathered evidence from different kinds of studies that discredit these and the many other claims of estrogen's dangers. Psychologist Carole Wade, a friend and co-author of Carol's, often used a homey example to explain scientific investigation to her college classes. "Accumulating facts to support an outdated theory in science," she said, "is like fitting a double-size sheet onto a queen-size mattress—you can get three corners to work but not the fourth. Some scientists will do everything they can to get that sheet to fit. But eventually they will need a new sheet or a new mattress." The "estrogen causes breast cancer" evidence has become a sheet that is not fitting the bed. But if you are in the double-size-sheet business, you're going to fight to get that fourth corner to work.

Cognitive psychologist Daniel Kahneman calls this protective mechanism "theory-induced blindness," a condition he has diagnosed in himself as well as in many of his colleagues and other scientists. "Once you have accepted a theory and used it as a tool in your thinking," he wrote, "it is extraordinarily difficult to notice its flaws. If you come upon an observation that does not seem to fit the model, you assume that there must be a perfectly good explanation that you are somehow missing. You give the theory the benefit of the doubt, trusting the community of experts who have accepted it."[10]

We are well aware that critics will accuse us of our own theory-induced blindness. They have two major criticisms of our arguments: first, that we must be biased by conflicts of interest, and second, that we are discounting the importance of the single most important study of hormone therapy, the randomized controlled trial conducted by the Women's Health Initiative.

Consumer activists and bioethicists have written extensively about the problem of conflicts of interest in research. (Carol has as well.[11]) John Ioannidis, now professor of medicine and of health research and policy at Stanford University School of Medicine, has long been a powerful, eloquent voice in criticizing research in medicine that is paid for by the pharmaceutical industry, and he includes the research on HRT in that category.[12] I respect his work and I know from personal correspondence with him that he believes that the data implicating hormones as a risk of breast cancer are strong and scientifically reliable. We have agreed to disagree about HRT. It's certainly true that researchers who accept funding from pharmaceutical companies are more likely to get the results that their funders want, but the problem of bias in interpreting a study's results afflicts many investigators, regardless of who is paying them. In a review of 164 randomized controlled studies related to breast cancer published between 1995 and 2011, researchers found that "spin and bias" in interpreting results were prevalent in a high percentage of them, and the source of funding (industry or government) made no difference.[13]

The lesson is not that all research is hopelessly tainted. It is that all humans are biased—sometimes by money, sometimes by personal convictions—and that we all must do our best to critically evaluate and weigh the best scientific and clinical information that we can get.

And now, one more time, the Women's Health Initiative.

Ten Key Problems with the Women's Health Initiative

In December 2017, the *Journal of the American Medical Association* published a report from the U.S. Preventive Services Task Force (USPSTF) that reiterated its opposition to hormone therapy for postmenopausal women who do not have bothersome symptoms. The review specified that it was not going to address the use of hormones for preventing or treating menopausal symptoms but adamantly advised against the use of ERT or HRT for the primary prevention of chronic conditions in postmenopausal women.[14] The report said that women taking estrogen alone had significantly lower risks of breast cancer, diabetes, and osteoporotic fractures than women taking placebo, but they had significantly higher risks of gallbladder disease, stroke, urinary incontinence, and venous blood clots. In addition, compared with women taking placebo, women taking combination HRT had significantly lower risks of colorectal cancer, diabetes, and osteoporotic fractures but significantly higher risks of breast cancer, dementia, gallbladder disease, stroke, urinary incontinence, and blood clots. Although the task force confirmed that HRT has many benefits, it concluded that the risks outweighed them.

The task force's conclusions were based almost entirely on the findings of the Women's Health Initiative. Deborah Grady, a respected researcher and epidemiologist, wrote the accompanying editorial:

> Twenty-five years ago, I coauthored a systematic review of the literature that supported guidelines from the American College of Physicians for counseling asymptomatic post-menopausal women about preventive HT [hormone therapy]. At the time, there were more than 30 studies supporting the benefits of HT for prevention of osteoporotic fractures and coronary disease events. The guidelines suggested that HT for prevention of disease should be considered by all women and recommended for women at risk for coronary heart disease. However, all of the studies included in the systematic review were observational. No randomized trials with clinical outcomes had been conducted.[15]

Grady, like the U.S. Preventive Services Task Force and many other groups that have based their practice guidelines on the Women's Health Initiative, places great confidence in the randomized controlled study. But as we showed in chapter 3, sometimes that gold standard has jagged edges and warped centers, and it is not the only path to truth; in many medical domains, observational studies produce findings of equally good quality and utility. We described research that compared RCTs and observational studies for nineteen varied medical treatments and found that the results were similar in most areas.

In fact, the official journal of the American Society of Clinical Oncology issued a research statement in 2017 underscoring the "untapped potential of observational research to inform clinical decision making," because observational studies can often answer questions that cannot or have not been answered by RCTs.[16] In a 2017 review article in the *New England Journal of Medicine*, Thomas R. Frieden, former director of the Centers for Disease Control and Prevention, compared RCTs with other methods, identifying their strengths and weaknesses. Some research methods, he wrote, are superior to RCTs and provide "valid evidence for clinical and public health action.... Elevating RCTs at the expense of other potentially highly valuable sources of data is counterproductive."[17]

That is why, in this book, we have drawn from a wide variety of studies to see the picture that emerges from the mosaic they create. Roger Lobo, professor of obstetrics and gynecology and fellowship director in the division of reproductive endocrinology at the Columbia College of Physicians and Surgeons, did the same for a 2017 medical review paper on HRT. He showed that the 20 to 40 percent reduction in mortality rates for women on HRT is consistent across all scientific methods: observational meta-analysis, RCTs, the WHI itself, a Cochrane meta-analysis of randomized trials, and observational studies.[18]

With Lobo's rebuttal to "we are the only and best study of the issue" stance of the WHI, we will summarize ten things about the Women's Health Initiative that we believe severely limit its claim to gold-standard science and the validity of its claims:

1. The WHI rushed into publication without most of the co-investigators even having seen, let alone approved, the final paper that was submitted to *JAMA*. It was fifteen years before one of those investigators published his blistering account of the violations of the scientific process and publication that the WHI and *JAMA* committed.

2. The WHI's finding that HRT increased the risk of breast cancer — the principal reason the study was halted prematurely — was not statistically significant. Yet a few of the WHI's primary investigators decided that breast cancer was such a worry for American women that it would be all right to "lower the bar" of statistical convention in this case. Press releases trumpeting the statistically nonsignificant increase in breast cancer preceded the distribution of the published journal, and that scare made its way around the world before the evidence got out of bed.

3. The study's sample was not representative of menopausal women; their average age was sixty-three. Yet the researchers had no qualms about generalizing their conclusions and recommendations to women entering menopause in their fifties.

4. The study's sample was not representative of healthy women. Nearly half were current or past smokers; more than a third had been treated for high blood pressure; fully 70 percent were seriously overweight or obese.

5. The study's findings were often inconsistent and contradictory. In 2002, the investigators reported a slight, nonsignificant increased risk of breast cancer, but only among women on HRT; in 2003, that risk was marginally significant; in 2006, that risk disappeared. Women taking only estrogen had no increased risk at first; three years later, being on ERT was associated with a *lower* risk of breast cancer.

6. Some of the WHI's claims were found only by data mining, a statistical practice that is widely held to be unacceptable in scientific analysis. Data mining means that if you get a finding you aren't satisfied with, you go back into the numbers and manipulate them until you get a finding you do like. For example, in that 2006 paper, instead of reporting that the risk of HRT had disappeared, which it had overall, the researchers changed the rules of their own analyses, retrospectively substratifying the sample until they got a smaller group they could say was at greater risk—a misleading interpretation.[19]

7. The WHI claimed that estrogen didn't even help alleviate menopausal symptoms, but given that they were not studying women in their fifties who were actually having menopausal symptoms, this conclusion was both meaningless and silly.

8. The WHI claimed that HRT increased the risk of heart problems, but that risk occurred only during the first year of treatment and only among women who were more than twenty years postmenopause. Five years following their initial publication, the WHI investigators revised their findings and concluded that women who started HRT in the first ten years following menopause in fact reduced their risk of coronary artery disease.

9.   In 2004, the WHI raised the alarm that estrogen increased the risk of strokes. As we saw in chapter 5, this concern did not come at the recommendation of the WHI's own data safety and monitoring board; it was generated by the same small group that had sounded the false alarm about breast cancer. Moreover, the WHI used an extremely broad definition of *stroke*—it included transient, subtle deficits that went away in a day or two with no aftermath. When an independent reanalysis controlled for the statistical manipulations that had appeared to indicate danger, the supposed increased risk of stroke vanished.

10. Many of the WHI investigators have continued to promote alternatives to HRT that they incorrectly maintain are just as effective in preventing certain conditions: bisphosphonates and calcium for osteoporosis, statins for heart disease, physical and mental workouts for Alzheimer's, and the familiar panacea, a "healthy diet" and exercise. But as we've seen, bisphosphonates and statins have their own side effects and are not as effective in the long term as hormones. The other suggestions are no better than placebos.

For these reasons and many others, the North American Menopause Society issued a 2017 position statement noting that "hormone therapy does not need to be routinely discontinued in women aged older than 60 or 65 years and can be considered for continuation beyond age 65 years for persistent vasomotor symptoms, quality of life issues, or prevention of osteoporosis after appropriate evaluation and counseling of benefits and risks.... There are no data to support routine discontinuation in women age 65 years."[20] This position statement was endorsed by the following groups:

Academy of Women's Health

American Association of Clinical Endocrinologists

American Association of Nurse Practitioners

American Medical Women's Association

American Society for Reproductive Medicine

Asociación Mexicana para el Estudio del Climaterio

Association of Reproductive Health Professionals

Australasian Menopause Society

British Menopause Society

Canadian Menopause Society

Chinese Menopause Society

Colegio Mexicano de Especialistas en Ginecologia y
    Obstetricia

Czech Menopause and Andropause Society

Dominican Menopause Society

European Menopause and Andropause Society

German Menopause Society

Groupe d'études de la ménopause et du vieillissement
    hormonal

Indian Menopause Society

International Menopause Society

International Osteoporosis Foundation

International Society for the Study of Women's Sexual Health

Israeli Menopause Society

Japan Society of Menopause and Women's Health

Korean Society of Menopause

Menopause Research Society of Singapore

National Association of Nurse Practitioners in Women's
    Health

Società Italiana della Menopausa
Society of Obstetricians and Gynaecologists of Canada
South African Menopause Society
Taiwanese Menopause Society
Thai Menopause Society

Reflections and Recommendations

Over the years, women have asked me many questions in my medical practice (not to mention at meetings, lectures, and dinner parties). Here are a few that come up frequently.

I didn't take hormones when I entered menopause. Can I start HRT in my sixties? At the age of sixty-three, a friend of mine who had never taken HRT called me. "Av," she said, "I've been listening to you talk about HRT for a long time, and I'd like to go on it. It's been six years since I entered menopause, and I've had no symptoms, but I'm concerned about my memory, my heart, and my sex life. Should I consider starting it now?"

It's a logical question. My position is that women who begin HRT during menopause for symptoms that seriously affect the quality of their lives have no reason not to take it for as long as it's beneficial and for as many years as they wish—under the guidance of their physicians, of course. But HRT isn't something a woman can start, stop, and resume every few years. It's not candy or a vitamin. There is a window of opportunity, roughly defined as the first ten years after a woman's last menstrual period, during which HRT has its greatest benefits. There may be an elevated risk for women who begin taking it more than ten years after menopause; if they have any preexisting atherosclerotic plaques, there is a risk of further obstructing an already narrowed artery, at least during the first year of HRT. This risk can be assessed with tests that determine arterial health and heart strength. I therefore encouraged my friend to have the tests; she passed with flying colors and began HRT. But I would not have been comfortable advising her to take hormones without that precaution.

What about the risks of HRT? Yes, there are risks. Most are minor, such as dry eyes (curiously, also a symptom of menopause itself).[21] Some women suffer migraine headaches during menstruation, and taking estrogen can lead to a return of those headaches when they enter menopause.[22] Some risks are more serious; as the U.S. Preventive Services Task Force noted, they include gallbladder disease and venous blood clots. But as Roger Lobo summarized, "Many of the adverse effects are not life-threatening and can be dealt with by adjusting the dose and preparation of HRT. These effects include breast tenderness, abdominal bloating, mood changes, uterine bleeding and an idiosyncratic elevation in blood pressure that might occur with oral oestrogens." He noted that more serious concerns such as venous thromboembolism (a blood clot in a vein that migrates to the lungs) might occur, but in healthy women entering menopause, "these risks are small or not significantly increased over placebo treatment.... The available data suggest no increased risks or serious adverse effects of HRT."[23] A growing number of professional organizations endorse Lobo's conclusions, regarding risks as being far outweighed by HRT's benefits for heart, bones, brain, and longevity. In 2013, the British Menopause Society and Women's Health Concern recommended that arbitrary limits should not be placed on how long women used HRT; if symptoms persisted, their statement noted, "the benefits of hormone therapy usually outweigh the risks."[24]

Aren't there other good ways of treating the symptoms of menopause? In chapter 2, we noted that menopausal symptoms may affect up to 80 percent of perimenopausal and postmenopausal women, and that these symptoms last an average of seven to twelve years. While most symptoms eventually clear with time, the symptoms associated with urogenital atrophy, including vaginal itching, urinary burning, urinary frequency, and painful sexual intercourse, become more pronounced as a woman grows older. These symptoms can often be treated successfully with topical estrogen creams.[25] Herbal remedies help about 20 percent of women, around the same success rate as any placebo. Neurontin, an anti-seizure medication, and Paxil, an antidepressant, reduce hot flashes in about 60 percent of women, but they do not help other menopausal symptoms, such as joint pains, insomnia, and heart palpitations. Of course, the search for successful nonhormonal treatments continues. In 2018, researchers at Imperial College London reported relief of hot flashes in women treated with a nonhormonal oral medication (neurokinin 3 receptor antagonist).[26] Their study was very small, only twenty-eight women, but it was a randomized controlled one, and larger studies will surely be done.

Can't I just take the lowest dose for the shortest time? As we saw in chapter 2, there is no scientific basis for this recommendation, although it still appears on all preparations of estrogen. It seems to have resulted from an uncomfortable compromise for the physicians who believed that hormones were dangerous but knew that they helped many women. The North American Menopause Society's position statement on HRT advises clinicians to move away from this simplistic advice and instead prescribe the dose and formulation that meet each patient's needs and concerns based on the woman's age, time of menopause, and any unique health risks she might have. The NAMS also agreed that there should be no "stop date" or mandatory limitation on length of time a woman takes HRT, and so did a 2010 scientific position paper from the Endocrine Society.[27]

I can't underscore this point strongly enough. As we have seen, for some conditions—notably osteoporosis and, most likely, cognitive decline—HRT's benefits stop when a woman stops taking it. A woman who had been in my breast cancer study told me that, after she'd been on HRT for ten years, her doctor suggested she go off it; there was no evidence, the doctor said, of any additional benefit. But that doctor was wrong. As we saw in chapter 4, when older women stop hormones, bone loss accelerates rapidly; after six years, they have the same degree of bone loss as women who have never taken hormones.

How should I think about my symptoms and decide if HRT is right for me? If you are in perimenopause or menopause and considering HRT as a way to improve your quality of life, begin by reviewing the symptoms listed at the start of chapter 2. Be sure to take note not only of familiar symptoms like hot flashes and night sweats but also those symptoms not usually associated with menopause, such as joint pain, heart palpitations, headaches, and insomnia. Ask yourself: "How severe is each symptom? How much does that symptom affect my quality of life (not at all, it's tolerable, it's pretty bad, or it's unbearable)?" When doctors or researchers try to assess a woman's quality of life by asking her for a vague overall summary—"How's your well-being, your mood, your health?"—

they generally evoke a woman's tendency to cope and not complain, and they don't get a true sense of whether any specific symptoms or concerns are troubling her.

Why not take statins instead of HRT to protect my heart? As we discussed in chapter 3, heart disease kills up to seven times as many women each year as breast cancer does (300,000 versus 41,000); in every decade of a woman's life after age thirty, heart disease is responsible for more deaths than breast cancer. Being on ERT or HRT can reduce the risk of acute cardiovascular events and death by up to 50 percent. Most medical organizations counsel against using hormones to protect heart health, instead advising statins to reduce cholesterol and anti-arrhythmia drugs to control palpitations. But statins do not reduce a woman's risk of having a *first* heart attack, and these drugs are not free from potentially serious side effects. Statins may cause diabetes or liver damage, and anti-arrhythmics may cause unacceptable slowing of the heart rate.

Why not take calcium and bisphosphonates to prevent osteoporosis and bone fractures? The number of female deaths annually in the United States associated with osteoporotic hip fractures is approximately the same as the number of deaths from breast cancer. As we saw in chapter 4, HRT and ERT reduce the risk of osteoporotic hip fractures by 30 to 50 percent, but women should remain on hormones for at least ten years to achieve this benefit; according to some experts, they should continue hormones indefinitely. While calcium and vitamin D may be helpful in strengthening bone to avoid hip fractures in premenopausal women who also exercise, they do not appear to be of any appreciable benefit in postmenopausal women who are not taking HRT. As we saw, a 2017 major review of thirty-three randomized trials found no associations between calcium, vitamin D, or combined calcium and vitamin D supplements and the incidence of nonvertebral, vertebral, or total fractures.[28] Bisphosphonates, whether taken by mouth or by injection, do decrease the risk of hip fractures at first, but, paradoxically, they increase the fracture risk after five years. In addition, they can cause stomach upset and, rarely, a serious and painful loss of bone in the jaw region. Evista (raloxifene) has been approved for the prevention of osteoporosis, but unlike estrogen, it has not been shown to affect the risk of hip fractures.

What about taking estradiol and other bioidenticals instead of Premarin? I am not comfortable with the whole "mares' urine" business. We addressed this widespread concern in chapter 2, but it bears repeating. *Bioidentical* refers to prescription hormones that have the same molecular structure as hormones that are naturally produced by the body. Adult women produce estradiol, the most prominent circulating estrogen, along with estriol and estrone. (*Bioidentical estrogen* usually refers to estradiol but it can also refer to estriol or estrone.) Premarin, the most commonly marketed form of estrogen, is extracted from pregnant mares' urine, a source that makes some women uncomfortable; however, it contains at least ten molecular forms of estrogen. Commercially manufactured estrogen and bioidentical estrogen (usually estradiol) are both approved and regulated by the FDA.

However, *compounded* bioidentical hormones, which are widely used in the United States, are generally prepared by a local pharmacy in response to a prescription written by a woman's physician. They are not standardized pharmaceutical products; they are not regulated by the FDA. That is why I, along with all major medical societies, discourage their use as an alternative to approved forms of estrogen and progesterone.[29]

Does the form of estrogen that I take make a difference? I realize that many women who are on HRT are taking estrogen in the form of a patch rather than as a pill, and they often ask me if that is okay. The reason they take estrogen in this form is usually that their gynecologists tell them that the patch is "not as harmful" in that it reduces the risk of clots. That is true, but what they don't add is that the patch is "not as helpful" either. Not all forms of estrogen have equal benefits on cognitive function, for example, or on reducing heart disease. The oral form appears to be more beneficial than the patch in preventing cardiovascular disease and stroke.[30] And Roberta Diaz Brinton and her colleagues, who have long been studying estrogen and brain function in relation to Alzheimer's, discovered that one form of estrogen that is found only in Premarin, called equilin, stimulates the growth of neurons in the cortex and other regions of the brain.[31]

What about exercise, mental and physical, to reduce my risk of dementia and cognitive decline? As we saw in chapter 5, for American women now age forty-five, at least 20 percent are projected to develop dementia during their remaining years, and half of those cases of dementia will be from Alzheimer's disease. A woman in her sixties is twice as likely to develop Alzheimer's as she is to develop breast cancer, and whereas deaths from heart disease, strokes, and breast cancer are falling, the number of deaths associated with Alzheimer's disease is steadily rising as the population ages. No nonhormonal treatment is effective in slowing or reversing the tragic symptoms of Alzheimer's and other dementias — not drugs, not mental exercises, not even physical workouts. The only successful intervention at present is hormone therapy, which decreases the risk of Alzheimer's in approximately 40 to 50 percent of the women who take it, especially if they have been doing so for at least ten years.

Is progesterone a problem? For many years, it was the use of estrogen that was believed to put postmenopausal women at increased risk of developing breast cancer. Now we are learning that that isn't so; estrogen might even decrease that risk. So attention turned to the possible harms of progesterone. When women take estrogen combined with natural, micronized progesterone, no increased risk of breast cancer has thus far been observed in any study. While I don't agree, some investigators believe there is a very small increased risk when the form of progesterone is synthetic progestin, but even so, it is no more than 2 percent. (See chapter 7.) And even if HRT increases the risk of breast cancer by this modest increment, recall that women on HRT live, on average, years longer than those not taking HRT.

I've had breast cancer but I'm now in menopause and having some terrible symptoms. Can I safely take HRT? Yes. (See chapter 6, and then talk to your doctor.)

The Process of Science and the Art of Medicine

Sir George White Pickering, a British medical doctor and professor of medicine at the University of Oxford, understood well the conflicting demands on every physician who seeks to help patients with the best available scientific information. "If you are a clinician," he said, "you must believe that you know what will help your patient; otherwise, you cannot counsel, you cannot prescribe. If you are a scientist, however, you must be uncertain—a scientist who no longer asks questions is a bad scientist."[32]

For me, the practice of medicine is like walking a tightrope, balancing between art and science, certainty and uncertainty—here's a drug or regimen that benefits patients overall, but some individuals will not do well on it. For any treatment, we physicians are always calculating whether the benefits outweigh the risks and wondering how that calculation might be customized for any given patient. Science, after all, gives us overall patterns and predictions for groups; it can't tell us what a particular individual should do. That's why smokers are forever pointing to their aunt Sally or great-uncle Morty who smoked three packs a day and lived to be ninety-nine; they rely on the outlying exception to justify smoking and ignore the more important statistic, namely the immense risk to their own health. Conversely, some women say, "My friend Harriet took HRT for five years and got breast cancer, so I'll never consider it." They are relying on an understandably compelling anecdote, but one that doesn't conform to the greater evidence. And if Harriet hadn't taken HRT, can we be sure she would not have gotten breast cancer? And if Harriet had drunk coffee every morning for five years and then got breast cancer, would that be a reason to forgo coffee?

I draw insight from the kitten study, which is rather like the neurological counterpart of Kahneman's notion of theory-induced blindness. Like human infants, kittens are born with the visual ability to detect horizontal and vertical lines and other spatial orientations. But if they are deprived of normal visual experience, these cells deteriorate and the cats' perception suffers. In one classic study, kittens were reared in darkness for five months after birth, but for several hours each day, they were put into a special cylinder that permitted them to see only vertical or horizontal lines. Later, the cats that had been exposed only to horizontal lines had trouble perceiving vertical ones; they would run to play with horizontal bars but not vertical bars.[33] Give them a chair, and they would jump onto its horizontal seat but repeatedly bump into its legs. Give the "vertical" kittens the same chair, and they would happily weave around its legs but literally not see the horizontal seat to curl up on.

I have often observed how mental blinders can prevent physicians and patients from seeing the whole picture. I understand why many people are distrustful of modern medicine, which often seems a coldhearted enterprise involving technology and medications administered by busy physicians who lack the time to focus on the human beings in front of them—the human beings who are full of uncertainty, worry, and fear. I understand why so many people today are drawn to alternative medicine, with its promises of "natural" remedies, "bioidentical" compounds, and humanistic concerns for the whole person. But just as a healthy kitten needs to perceive the legs *and* the seat of that chair, a single perception on its own distorts one's field of vision.

I see my patients as being far more than the immediate problem they come in with; I temper what I've learned from science with what I've learned about human beings. Like all oncologists, I am fully aware of the toll that breast cancer exacts on women, their loved ones, and the general population. But I do not want that concern to dominate my advice or plan of treatment for any given woman. Some HRT researchers and breast cancer activists are like the vertical-line kittens, able to focus only on breast cancer and their patients' fear of breast cancer; breast cancer is *all* they fear and all they see. But this focus can lead to a failure to consider women's greater risk of suffering from heart disease and osteoporosis, conditions that are far more likely to be fatal. A diagnosis of breast cancer is no longer inevitably a death sentence, and it hasn't been for decades. Successful treatment most often no longer requires a mastectomy; the majority of patients are now treated without chemotherapy; and, as I keep repeating, 90 percent or more of women diagnosed with early breast cancer today are likely to be cured. The patient's life situation, symptoms, risk of other illnesses, and personal goals must be factored into any recommendations for taking ERT or HRT, as should the form, dose, and duration of that treatment.

For that reason, I would never presume to advise readers of a book—even this one—of their best or healthiest course of action. Nevertheless, as someone who has spent his life walking that tightrope between science and practice, I am convinced of the immense benefits of HRT, including its likely ability to prolong women's lives. For women's health and quality of life, for better science and medical practice, it's time to retire outdated beliefs about estrogen. Women should not be taking HRT because of Robert Wilson's impossible and patronizing notion that it will make them "feminine forever." But, as Bernadine Healy advised so many years ago, it is likely to make them healthier longer. That's why there's no question in my mind that estrogen matters.

Afterword

S ince this book was published we have continued to gather evidence about estrogen's benefits, and we attend closely to any studies that question our conclusions. We provide details of new findings and references on the update page of the book's website (https://estrogenmatters.com/), but here are some highlights.

First and foremost, the WHI has walked back virtually all of their early alarmist findings. In recent publications, they reported that estrogen does not increase "all-cause mortality" or deaths from heart disease and cancer. Actually, they said, it increases longevity, most notably when begun within ten years of the last menstrual period. It is the best preventative for osteoporotic hip fracture. It is safe and effective when applied vaginally for local symptoms. And, in the most striking about-face from their 2003 headlines that HRT "did not have a clinically meaningful effect on health-related quality of life" for women in menopause, they stated in 2019 that "Hormone therapy is the most effective treatment for managing menopausal vasomotor symptoms."[1] *Now* they write that "hot flashes and night sweats affect approximately 70% of midlife women and may persist for a decade or longer," having significant adverse effects "on sleep, daily functioning, and quality of life."

And, by the way, they add that "cognitive and mood symptoms often accompany disruptive hot flashes." For these reasons, women with frequent, severe menopausal symptoms "may greatly benefit from hormone therapy." Better late than never, but earlier would have been better for the countless thousands of women the WHI deprived of the "most effective" treatment.

As for women's deep-seated fears of breast cancer as their main reason to avoid estrogen, in 2020 the WHI investigators reported a 23% *decreased* incidence of breast cancer among women randomized to estrogen — after nineteen years of follow-up. It's the combination of estrogen and progesterone (HRT), they still maintained, that raises the risk.[2] But two medical sleuths challenged that finding, reporting it was due to a statistical misinterpretation: The women on HRT did not have an *increased* risk; the control group had a *reduced* risk, because many of the women in that group had been on estrogen before the study! When they were removed from analysis, the supposed increased risk of HRT vanished.[3]

And what about the WHI's frightening claim that HRT increases women's risk of death from breast cancer? They have withdrawn that claim, too. In 2021, a WHI principal investigator reported that after twenty years of follow-up, women randomized to the combination of estrogen and progesterone had no statistically significant increase in breast cancer mortality, while women randomized to estrogen alone had a 40% reduced risk of death from breast cancer.[4]

Even more good news for the many women concerned about the safety of pregnancy, when estrogen rises tenfold, following breast cancer: A collaborative study from research institutions around the world concluded that pregnancy following treatment of breast cancer had no negative effect on prognosis, regardless of estrogen receptor assay positivity, after a median follow-up of 7.2 years. And a retrospective international cohort study of 1,252 breast cancer patients with BRCA mutations, published in 2020, reported no increased risk of breast cancer recurrence associated with pregnancy following treatment.[5]

Nonetheless, as of this writing in 2021, we have yet to see an NIH press conference convened to reassure women of the benefits of estrogen and publicly explain what was wrong with the original WHI scare stories that many doctors still hold as gospel. On the contrary, whenever someone manages to assemble yet another huge vat of numbers and pull out a tiny but spurious "finding" that can alarm women, headlines follow like a dog after a biscuit. In 2019, the prestigious British journal *The Lancet* published a paper claiming that HRT increases the risk of breast cancer, generating the inevitable headlines and fears, and so we scrutinized it closely. Once again, the data did not support the alarm.[6]

We are still waiting for that press conference.

Acknowledgments

From Avrum

The first person I want to thank is Carol. During the course of our long friendship, we have co-authored scientific papers, editorials, and book reviews, and, knowing the long-standing importance of this issue to me and for women's health, she set her sights on helping me write this book. It is her persistence, her insights, her merciless critical appraisals, her sense of humor, and her talent as a writer that brought this book to life.

It can be daunting to hold and espouse a minority opinion in medicine, but I never felt alone. I am grateful to Phil DiSaia, former president of the American Board of Obstetrics and Gynecology and professor in the School of Medicine at UC Irvine, who wrote about the benefits and risks of HRT years before I did, published one of the earliest studies of HRT administered to breast cancer survivors, and has always supported my efforts in this area. Other physicians who have helped me both by example and with advice are Roger Lobo, Basil Stoll, Rena Vassilopoulou-Sellin, and Dietrich von Fournier. I also wish to thank the physicians across diverse specialties who offered encouragement and counsel, notably Michael Baum, Jonathan Berek, David Decker, Marc Espie, Faith

Fitzgerald, and John Stevenson, along with colleagues and friends who read earlier versions of this argument and provided many helpful suggestions: Judy Baldwin, Peter Clarke, Susan Evans, Patricia T. Kelly, Nancy Reaven, and Carole Wade.

I am deeply grateful to the many members of the Los Angeles medical community, most especially those affiliated with the Tarzana Regional Medical Center, at which I served as director of oncology, chief of staff, and director of continuing medical education. These colleagues listened patiently to my opinions and encouraged my continued study of HRT for breast cancer survivors. Among the many people who made it possible for me to swim upstream by publishing my ideas in professional journals or giving me a public forum for debate are Edward Bouwer, Ken Frazier, Phyllis Greenberger, Val Jones, Michael J. Mastrangelo, Michael Mosher, Saar Porrath, Nancy Raymon, Erik Rifkin, Selma Schimmel, Mel Silverstein, and Steven Strauss. My special thanks to Vince DeVita, editor in chief of the *Cancer Journal,* who spent Christmas Eve reading Carol's and my first paper on HRT and who called the next morning to say he had recommended it be published.

Finally, warm thanks to N. J. Nakamura, the oncology nurse-practitioner in my office who was our study coordinator, and Pamela J. Gay, research librarian at Providence Holy Cross Medical Center, who provided citations and full text papers within hours of every request.

From Avrum and Carol
We want to express our gratitude to Jane Isay, the much-admired book editor and publisher with whom Carol once worked. Over

lunch in New York, listening to Carol talk about Avrum's work, Jane nearly dropped her fork. "It's a book!" she exclaimed. "A medical mystery story— *Who Killed HRT?*" That title didn't survive the conversation, but the idea did. In a heartbeat Jane introduced us to Gail Ross, head of the Ross Yoon agency, who became our literary agent as soon as she learned about our project. In a world full of people grousing about their agents, we could not be more pleased by our experience working with Gail and her staff, especially Dara Kaye, who did superb editing on our initial book proposal. Gail took on our project with alacrity and has remained an enthusiastic supporter and adviser. She got us to Tracy Behar, publisher and editor in chief of Little, Brown Spark, who introduced herself by saying, "I am your ideal reader." And she has been—and our ideal editor as well. She raised important conceptual concerns, caught points that were unclear, and, being as knowledgeable about scientific methods as she is, never pressed us to sacrifice evidence for the sake of making the book more "pop medicine." We have had a superb experience with everyone we have worked with: associate editor Ian Straus, Tracy's witty and efficient associate, who never dropped a detail; executive production editor Peggy Freudenthal, who so expertly steered the manuscript through the shoals of production; associate art director Lucy Kim, who designed the elegant cover; Tracy Roe, the undisputed queen of copyediting, whose close and informed reading enhanced and clarified the text; and the meticulous, superb work of our exceptional proofreader, Barbara Jatkola. Our warmest thanks to the entire Little, Brown team for making the experience of writing this book so gratifying and pleasurable.

Notes

Introduction: Who Killed HRT?

1. P. T. Kelly, *Assess Your True Risk of Breast Cancer* (New York: Henry Holt, 2000).
2. Goldman L, Tosteson AN. Uncertainty about postmenopausal estrogen: Time for action, not debate. N Engl J Med. 1991;325:800–802.
3. Weiss NS, Ure CL, Ballard JH, et al. Decreased risk of fractures of the hip and lower forearm with postmenopausal use of estrogen. N Engl J Med. 1980;303:1195–98.

   Kiel DP, Felson DT, Anderson JJ, et al. Hip fracture and the use of estrogens in postmenopausal women: The Framingham study. N Engl J Med. 1987;317:1169–74.
4. Col NF, Eckman MH, Karas RH, et al. Patient-specific decisions about hormone replacement therapy in postmenopausal women. JAMA. 1997;277:1140–47.
5. B. Healy, *A New Prescription for Women's Health: Getting the Best Medical Care in a Man's World* (New York: Viking, 1995), 200–201.
6. Clarke RB, Howell A, Potten CS, Anderson E. Dissociation between steroid receptor expression and cell proliferation in the human breast. Cancer Res. 1997;57:4987–91. We realize that this is a complex matter; see also Sleeman KE, Kendrick H, Robertson D, et al. Dissociation of estrogen receptor expression and in vivo stem cell activity in the mammary gland. J Cell Biol. 2007;176:19–26.

7. Bluming AZ, Tavris C. Hormone replacement therapy: Real concerns and false alarms. Cancer J. 2009;15:93–104.

   Bluming AZ, Tavris C. What are the real risks for breast cancer? Climacteric. 2012;15:133–38.

   Bluming AZ, Tavris C. Chains of evidence, mosaics of data: Does estrogen *cause* breast cancer? How would we know? Climacteric. 2012;15:531–37.

Chapter 1: Does Estrogen Cause Breast Cancer?

1. R. P. Feynman, *The Meaning of It All: Thoughts of a Citizen Scientist* (Reading, MA: Perseus, 1998), 71.
2. Love RR, Philips J. Oophorectomy for breast cancer: History revisited. J Natl Cancer Inst. 2002;94:1433–34.
3. R. A. Wilson, *Feminine Forever* (New York: Pocket Books, 1966).
4. G. Kolata and M. Petersen, "Hormone Replacement Study a Shock to the Medical System," *New York Times,* July 10, 2002.
5. Smith DC, Prentice R, Thompson DJ, et al. Association of exogenous estrogen and endometrial carcinoma. N Engl J Med. 1975;293:1164–67.

   Mack TM, Pike MC, Henderson BE, et al. Estrogen and endometrial cancer in a retirement community. N Engl J Med. 1976;294:1262–67.

   Ziel HK, Kinkle WD. Increased risk of endometrial carcinoma among users of conjugated estrogens. N Engl J Med. 1975;293:1167–70.
6. Gambrell RD. Prevention of endometrial cancer with progestogens. Maturitas. 1986;8:159–68.
7. Brinton LA, Hoover R, and Fraumeni JF. Menopausal oestrogens and breast cancer risk: An expanded case-control study. Br J Cancer. 1986;54:825–32.
8. Armstrong BK. Estrogen therapy after the menopause: Boon or bane? Med J Aust. 1988;148:213–14.

9. Palmer JR, Rosenberg L, Clark EA, et al. Breast cancer risk after estrogen replacement therapy: Results from the Toronto breast cancer study. Am J Epidemiol. 1991;134:1386–95.

10. Dupont WD, Page DL. Menopausal estrogen replacement therapy and breast cancer. Arch Intern Med. 1991;151:67–72.

11. Nachtigall MJ, Smilen SW, Nachtigall RD, et al. Incidence of breast cancer in a 22-year study of women receiving estrogen-progestin replacement therapy. Obstet Gynecol. 1992;80:827–30.

12. Dupont WD, Page DL, Rogers LW, et al. Influence of exogenous estrogens, proliferative breast disease, and other variables on breast cancer risk. Cancer. 1989;63:948–57.

    Dupont WD, Page DL, Parl FF, et al. Estrogen replacement therapy in women with a history of proliferative breast disease. Cancer. 1999;85:1277–83.

13. Consensus Development Conference: Prophylaxis and treatment of osteoporosis. BMJ. 1987;295:914–15.

14. Martin KA, Freeman MW. Postmenopausal hormone replacement therapy. N Engl J Med. 1993;328:1115–17.

15. Stanford JL, Weiss NS, Voight LF, et al. Combined estrogen and progestin hormone replacement therapy in relation to risk of breast cancer in middle-aged women. JAMA. 1995;274:137–42.

16. Colditz GA, Hankinson SE, Hunter DJ, et al. The use of estrogens and progestins and the risk of breast cancer in postmenopausal women. N Engl J Med. 1995;332:1589–93.

17. Willis DB, Calle EE, Miracle-McMahill HL, et al. Estrogen replacement therapy and risk of fatal breast cancer in a prospective cohort of postmenopausal women in the United States. Cancer Causes Control. 1996;7:449–57.

18. Col NF, Eckman MH, Karas RH, et al. Patient-specific decisions about hormone replacement therapy in postmenopausal women. JAMA. 1997;277:1140–47.

19. Sellers TA, Mink PJ, Ceerhan JR, et al. The role of hormone replacement therapy and the risk for breast cancer and total mortality in

women with a family history of breast cancer. Ann Intern Med. 1997;127:973–80.

20. Takeuchi M, Saeki T, Sano M, et al. Case-control study of hormone replacement therapy (HRT) and breast cancer in Japanese women. Proc ASCO. 2006;24:10012.

21. Stefanick ML, Anderson GL, Margolis KL, et al. Effects of conjugated equine estrogens on breast cancer and mammography screening in postmenopausal women with hysterectomy. JAMA. 2006;295:1647–57.

22. Rebbeck TR, Levin AM, Eisen A, et al. Breast cancer risk after bilateral prophylactic oophorectomy in BRCA1 mutation carriers. J Natl Cancer Inst. 1999;91:1475–79.

    Rebbeck TR, Friebel T, Wagner T, et al. Effect of short-term hormone replacement therapy on breast cancer risk reduction after bilateral prophylactic oophorectomy in BRCA1 and BRCA2 mutation carriers: The PROSE Study Group. J Clin Oncol. 2005;23:7804–10.

23. Eisen A, Lubinski J, Gronwald J, et al. Hormone therapy and the risk of breast cancer in BRCA1 mutation carriers. J Natl Cancer Inst. 2008;100:1361–67.

24. Kotsopoulos J, Huzarski T, Gronwald J, et al. Hormone replacement therapy after menopause and risk of breast cancer in BRCA1 mutation carriers: A case-control study. Breast Cancer Res Treat. 2016;155:365–73.

25. Bergkvist L, Adami HO, Persson I, et al. The risk of breast cancer after estrogen and estrogen-progestin replacement. N Engl J Med. 1989;321:393–97.

26. Bergkvist L, Adami HO, Persson I, et al. Prognosis after breast cancer diagnosis in women exposed to estrogens and estrogen-progesterone replacement therapy. Am J Epidemiol. 1989;130:221–28.

27. Barrett-Connor E. Postmenopausal estrogen replacement and breast cancer. N Engl J Med. 1989;321:319–20.

28. Estrogen replacement and breast cancer. Harvard Medical School Health Letter. 1989;14(12):1–3.

29. Collaborative Group on Hormonal Factors in Breast Cancer. Breast cancer and hormone replacement therapy: Collaborative reanalysis of data from 51 epidemiological studies of 52,705 women with breast cancer and 108,411 women without breast cancer. Lancet. 1997;350:1047–59.

30. Shapiro S, Farmer RDT, Seaman H, et al. Does hormone replacement therapy cause breast cancer? An application of causal principles to three studies. Part 1. The Collaborative Reanalysis. J Fam Plann Reprod Health Care. 2011;37:103–9.

31. Rossouw JE, Anderson GL, Prentice RL, et al. Risks and benefits of estrogen plus progestin in healthy postmenopausal women: Principal results from the Women's Health Initiative Randomized Controlled Trial. JAMA. 2002;288:321–33.

32. Ettinger B, Wang SM, Leslie RS, et al. Evolution of postmenopausal hormone therapy between 2002 and 2009. Menopause. 2012;19:610–15.

33. Anderson G. Release of the results of the Estrogen Plus Progestin Trial of the WHI: Data and Safety Monitoring. Press conference remarks. WHI Coordinating Center, July 9, 2002.

34. Chlebowski RT, Hendrix SL, Langer RD, et al. for the WHI investigators. Influence of estrogen plus progestin on breast cancer and mammography in healthy postmenopausal women: The Women's Health Initiative Randomized Trial. JAMA. 2003;289:3243–53.

35. Anderson GL, Chlebowski RT, Rossouw JE, et al. Prior hormone therapy and breast cancer risk in the Women's Health Initiative randomized trial of estrogen plus progestin. Maturitas. 2006;55: 103–15. Nevertheless, they did extract a small increased risk by mining their data and looking just at women who were randomized to be given HRT and who had taken HRT before entering the study. Later in this chapter we explain why trying to evoke a credible finding this way is scientifically unacceptable.

36. T. Parker-Pope, *The Hormone Decision* (Emmaus, PA: Rodale, 2007), 14.

37. Heiss G, Wallace R, Anderson GL, et al. Health risks and benefits three years after stopping randomized treatment with estrogen and progestin. JAMA. 2008;299:1036–45.

38. Chlebowski RT, Anderson GL, Gass M, et al. Estrogen plus progestin and breast cancer incidence and mortality in postmenopausal women. JAMA. 2010;304:1684–92.

39. Burger H. Hormone replacement therapy in the post–Women's Health Initiative era. Climacteric. 2003;6:11–36.

Genazzani AR, Gambacciani M. A personal initiative for women's health: To challenge the Women's Health Initiative. Gynecol Endocrinol. 2002;16:255–57.

Lemay A. The relevance of the Women's Health Initiative results on combined hormone replacement therapy and clinical practice. J Obstet Gynaecol Can. 2002;24:711–15.

40. Shapiro S, de Villers TJ, Pines A, et al. Risks and benefits of hormone therapy: Has medical dogma now been overturned? Climacteric. 2014;17:215–22.

See also Shapiro S. Risks of estrogen plus progestin therapy: A sensitivity analysis of the findings in the Women's Health Initiative randomized controlled trial. Climacteric. 2003;6:302–10. Although the WHI was reportedly a double-blind study (meaning that neither the patients nor the investigators knew who was receiving hormones and who was receiving placebo), 44.4 percent of the women given HRT and only 6.8 percent of the women taking the placebo pills were aware of the treatment they were receiving.

41. Langer RD. The evidence base for HRT: What can we believe? Climacteric. 2017;20:91–96.

42. Parker-Pope, *The Hormone Decision*, 12. The quote is Parker-Pope's report of what Rossouw told her; *high impact* was his term.

43. Rossouw JE. Estrogens for prevention of coronary heart disease: Putting the brakes on the bandwagon. Circulation. 1996;94:2982–85.

44. Beral V, Million Women Study Collaborators. Breast cancer and hormone-replacement therapy in the Million Women Study. Lancet. 2003;362:419–27.

45. G. Taubes, "Do We Really Know What Makes Us Healthy?," *New York Times Sunday Magazine*, September 16, 2007.

46. Asilomar Working Group on Recommendations for Reporting of Clinical Trials in the Biomedical Literature. Checklist of information for inclusion in reports of clinical trials. Ann Intern Med. 1996;124:741–43.

    Altman DG, Schulz KF, Moher D, et al. The revised CONSORT statement for reporting randomized trials: Explanation and elaboration. Ann Intern Med. 2001;134:663–94.

    Moher D, Schulz KF, Altman D for the CONSORT Group. The CONSORT statement: Revised recommendations for improving the quality of reports of parallel-group randomized trials. JAMA. 2001;285:1987–91.

    Gigerenzer G, Gaissmaier W, Kurz-Milcke E, et al. Helping doctors and patients make sense of health statistics. Psychol Sci Public Interest. 2008;8:53–96.

47. Individual references for each entry may be found in Bluming AZ, Tavris C. Hormone replacement therapy: Real concerns and false alarms. Cancer J. 2009;15:93–104; and Bluming AZ, Tavris C. What are the real risks for breast cancer? Climacteric. 2012;15: 133–38.

48. P. Bernstein, *Against the Gods: The Remarkable Story of Risk* (New York: John Wiley, 1996), 161.

49. Keating C. The social history of ISIS-2: Triumph and the path not taken. Lancet. 2015;386:e4–e5.

50. ISIS-2 (Second International Study of Infarct Survival) Collaborative Group. Aspirin's effect on myocardial infarct mortality: Randomized trial of intravenous streptokinase, oral aspirin, both or neither among 17,187 cases of suspected acute myocardial infarction. Lancet. 1988;2:349–60.

51. Sleight P. Debate: Subgroup analyses in clinical trials: Fun to look at—but don't believe them! Curr Control Trials Cardiovasc Med. 2000;1:25–27.

52. Colditz GA, Hankinson SE, Hunter DJ, et al. The use of estrogens and progestins and the risk of breast cancer in postmenopausal women. N Engl J Med. 1995;332:1589–93.

53. Schairer C, Lubin J, Troisi R, et al. Menopausal estrogen and estrogen-progestin replacement therapy and breast cancer risk. JAMA. 2000;283:485–91.

54. Santen RJ, Pinkerton J, McCartney C, et al. Risk of breast cancer with progestins in combination with estrogen as hormone replacement therapy. J Clin Endocrinol Metab. 2001;86:16–23.

55. Henderson BE, Paganini-Hill A, Ross RK. Decreased mortality in users of estrogen replacement therapy. Arch Intern Med. 1991;151: 75–78.

    Grodstein F, Stampfer MJ, Colditz GA, et al. Postmenopausal hormone therapy and mortality. N Engl J Med. 1997;336: 1769–75.

56. Susser M. What is a cause and how do we know one? A grammar for pragmatic epidemiology. Am J Epidemiol. 1991;133:635–48.

57. Taubes G. Epidemiology faces its limits. Science. 1995;269: 164–69.

58. For one study among very many, see Madsen KM, Hviid A, Vestergaard M, et al. A population-based study of measles, mumps, and rubella vaccination and autism. N Engl J Med. 2002;347: 1477–82. For the larger story of the vaccine hysteria, see S. Mnookin, *The Panic Virus: A True Story of Medicine, Science, and Fear* (New York: Simon and Schuster, 2011).

59. Charlton BG. Second thoughts: Attribution of causation in epidemiology: Chain or mosaic? J Clin Epidemiol. 1996;49:105–7.

60. Hill AB. The environment and disease: Association or causation? Proc R Soc Med. 1965;58:295–300.

61. Bush TL, Whiteman M, Flaws JA. Hormone replacement therapy and breast cancer: A qualitative review. Obstet Gynecol. 2001;98: 498–508.

62. Henderson IC. Risk factors for breast cancer development. Cancer. 1993;71:2127–40.

    Jemal A, Siegel R, Xu J, et al. Cancer statistics, 2010. CA: Cancer J Clin. 2010;60:277–300.

    Madigan M, Ziegler R, Benichou C, et al. Proportion of breast cancer cases in the United States explained by well-established risk factors. J Natl Cancer Inst. 1995;87:1681–85.

63. P. T. Kelly, *Assess Your True Risk of Breast Cancer* (New York: Henry Holt, 2000).

64. Haddow A, Watkinson JM, Paterson E. Influence of synthetic oestrogens upon advanced malignant disease. BMJ. 1944;2:393–98.

65. Massidda B, Mascia V, Broccia G, et al. Estrogen therapy of advanced breast cancer. Minerva Med. 1977;68:2509–16.

66. Mahtani RL, Stein A, Vogel CL. High-dose estrogen as salvage hormonal therapy for highly refractory metastatic breast cancer: A retrospective chart review. Clin Therap. 2009;31:2371–78.

67. Hortobagyi GN, Hug V, Buzdar AU, et al. Sequential cyclic combined hormonal therapy for metastatic breast cancer. Cancer. 1989;64:1002–6.

68. Ingle J, Ahmann D, Green S, et al. Randomized clinical trial of diethylstilbestrol versus tamoxifen in postmenopausal women with advanced breast cancer. N Engl J Med. 1981;304:16–21.

    Peethambaram P, Ingle J, Suman V, et al. Randomized clinical trial of diethylstilbestrol versus tamoxifen in postmenopausal women with metastatic breast cancer: An updated analysis. Breast Cancer Res Treat. 1999;54:117–22.

69. Lønning PE, Taylor PD, Anker G, et al. High-dose estrogen treatment in postmenopausal breast cancer patients heavily exposed to endocrine therapy. Breast Cancer Res Treat. 2001;67:111–16.

70. Craig Jordan V, Lewis-Wambi J, Kim H, et al. Exploiting the apoptotic actions of oestrogen to reverse anti-hormonal drug resistance in oestrogen receptor positive breast cancer patients. Breast. 2007;16(Suppl 2):105–13.

71. Zahl P-H, Mæhlen J. A decline in breast-cancer incidence. Letter to the editor. N Engl J Med. 2007;357:509–13.

72. Ravdin PM, Cronin KA, Howlander N, et al. The decrease in breast cancer incidence in 2003 in the United States. Reply. N Engl J Med. 2007;356:1670–74.

73. Bluming AZ. A decline in breast-cancer incidence. Letter to the editor. N Engl J Med. 2007;357:509. (See chapter 8.)

74. S. Mukherjee, *The Emperor of All Maladies: A Biography of Cancer* (New York: Scribner, 2010), 266.

75. Siegel RL, Miller KD, Jemal A. Cancer statistics, 2018. CA: Cancer J Clin. 2018;68:7–30.

76. Thun MJ, Hannan LM, Adams-Campbell LL, et al. Lung cancer occurrence in never-smokers: An analysis of 13 cohorts and 22 cancer registry studies. PLoS Med. 2008;5:e185.

    Fletcher AS, Erbas B, Kavanagh AM, et al. Use of hormone replacement therapy (HRT) and survival following breast cancer diagnosis. Breast. 2005;14:192–200.

    Miller KD, Siegel RL, Lin CC, et al. Cancer treatment and survivorship statistics, 2016. CA: Cancer J Clin. 2016;66:271–89.

77. Hoover R. Hormones in breast cancer: Etiology versus ideology. May 15, 2007; http://videocast.nih.gov/Summary.asp?File=13823.

Chapter 2: The "Change of Life" and the Quality of Life

1. *O, The Oprah Magazine,* August 2002; http://www.oprah.com/omagazine/be-aware-for-perimenopause/all.

2. S. T. Loh, *The Madwoman in the Volvo* (New York: W. W. Norton, 2014), 15.

3. T. Parker-Pope, *The Hormone Decision* (Emmaus, PA: Rodale, 2007), 133.

4. Utian WH, Gass ML, Pickar JH. Body mass index does not influence response to treatment, nor does body weight change with lower doses of conjugated estrogens and medroxyprogesterone acetate in early postmenopausal women. Menopause. 2004;11:306–14.

   Barnabei VM, Cochrane BB, Aragaki AK, et al. Menopausal symptoms and treatment-related effects of estrogen and progestin in the Women's Health Initiative. Obstet Gynecol. 2005;105: 1063–73.

5. E. S. Watkins, *The Estrogen Elixir: A History of Hormone Replacement Therapy in America* (Baltimore: Johns Hopkins University Press, 2007), 1.

6. Marriott LK, Wenk GL. Neurobiological consequences of long-term estrogen therapy. Curr Dir Psychol Sci. 2004;13:173–76.

7. Watkins, *The Estrogen Elixir,* 185.

8. Ibid.

9. G. Kolata, "Hormone Therapy, Already Found to Have Risks, Is Now Said to Lack Benefits," *New York Times,* March 18, 2003.

10. Nachtigall L. Treatment of estrogen deficiency symptoms in women surviving breast cancer. Part 4. Urogenital atrophy, vasomotor instability, sleep disorders, and related symptoms. Oncol. 1999;13:551–75.

11. G. N. Grob and A. V. Horwitz, *Diagnosis, Therapy, and Evidence: Conundrums in Modern American Medicine* (New Brunswick, NJ: Rutgers University Press, 2010), 195.

12. E. Martin, *The Woman in the Body: A Cultural Analysis of Reproduction* (Boston: Beacon, 1987).

13. S. Blaffer Hrdy, *Mother Nature: Maternal Instincts and How They Shape the Human Species* (New York: Ballantine, 1999).

    Pavelka, MSM, Fedigan LM. Menopause: A comparative life history perspective. Am J Phys Anthropol. 1991;34:13–38.

14. Avis NE, Crawford SL, Greendale G, et al. Duration of menopausal vasomotor symptoms over the menopause transition. JAMA Intern Med. 2015;175:531–39.

For commentary and review, see Judge DE. And the heat goes on. N Engl J Med. March 10, 2015.

15. Hays J, Ockene JK, Brunner RL, et al. Effects of estrogen plus progestin on health-related quality of life. N Engl J Med. 2003; 348:1839–54.

16. Ibid., 1839.

17. Watkins, *The Estrogen Elixir*, 1.

18. Nelson HD. Commonly used types of postmenopausal estrogen for treatment of hot flashes: Scientific review. JAMA. 2004;291: 1610–20.

19. ACOG Practice Bulletin No. 141: Management of menopausal symptoms. Obstet Gynecol. 2014;123:202–16.

   The North American Menopause Society has concurred in both its 2015 and 2017 position papers; see Gass ML, Maki PM, Shifren JL, et al. NAMS (North American Menopause Society) supports judicious use of systemic hormone therapy for women aged 65 years and older. Menopause. 2015;22:685–86; and the 2017 hormone therapy position statement of the North American Menopause Society. Menopause. 2017;24:728–53.

20. Welton AJ, Vickers MR, Kim J, et al. Health-related quality of life after combined hormone replacement therapy: Randomized controlled trial. BMJ. 2008;337:a1190.

21. Ockene JK, Barad DH, Cochrane BB, et al. Symptom experience after discontinuing use of estrogen plus progestin. JAMA. 2005; 294:183–93.

22. Christgau S, Tanko LB, Cloos PA, et al. Suppression of elevated cartilage turnover in postmenopausal women and in ovariectomized rats by estrogen and a selective estrogen-receptor modulator (SERM). Menopause. 2004;11:508–18.

23. Schmidt PJ, Nieman L, Danaceau MA, et al. Estrogen replacement in perimenopause-related depression: A preliminary report. Am J Obstet Gynecol. 2000;183:414–20.

Soares CN, Almeida OP, Joffe H, et al. Efficacy of estradiol for the treatment of depressive disorders in perimenopausal women: a double-blind, randomized, placebo-controlled trial. Arch Gen Psychiatry. 2001;58:529–34.

For a review, see Lobo RA, Bélisle S, Creasman WT, et al. Should symptomatic menopausal women be offered hormone therapy? Med Gen Med. 2006;8:40.

24. Kirsch I. Antidepressants and the placebo effect. Z Psychol [in English]. 2014;222:128–34.

25. K. Taylor, "Finding the Positive Side of Menopause," *Jewish Chronicle,* May 12, 2007; https://www.pressreader.com/uk/the -jewish-chronicle/20170512/282127816396074.

26. Couzi RJ, Helzsouer KJ, Fetting JH. Prevalence of menopausal symptoms among women with a history of breast cancer and attitudes toward estrogen replacement therapy. J Clin Oncol. 1995; 13:2737–44.

27. Hershman DL, Cho C, Crew KD. Management of complications from estrogen deprivation in breast cancer patients. Curr Oncol Rep. 2009;11:29–36.

28. Antoine C, Vandromme J, Fastrez M, et al. A survey among breast cancer survivors: Treatment of the climacteric after breast cancer. Climacteric. 2008;11:322–28.

29. Garrido-Oyarzún MF, Castelo-Branco C. Use of hormone therapy for menopausal symptoms and quality of life in breast cancer survivors: Safe and ethical? Gynecol Endocrinol. 2017;33: 10–15.

30. The 2017 hormone therapy position statement of the North American Menopause Society. Menopause. 2017;24:728–53.

31. Langer RD, Manson JE, Allison MA. Have we come full circle — or moved forward? The Women's Health Initiative 10 years on. Climacteric. 2012;15:206–12.

Utian WH. A decade post WHI, menopausal hormone therapy

comes full circle—need for independent commission. Climacteric. 2012;15:320–25.

32. C. Smyth, "Women Told Hormone Replacement Therapy Does Not Lead to Early Death," *Times* (UK), September 13, 2017; https://www.thetimes.co.uk/article/women-told-hrt-does-not-lead-to-early-death-ztk08tn7j?shareToken=ad8acbab104dce49546d8e90d85b7987.

33. Richard-Davis G, Manson JE. Vasomotor symptom duration in midlife women—research overturns dogma. JAMA Intern Med. 2015;175:540–41.

34. Santen RJ, Stuenkel CA, Davis SR, et al. Managing menopausal symptoms and associated clinical issues in breast cancer survivors. J Clin Endocrinol Metab. 2017;102:3647–61; https://doi.org/10.1210/jc.2017-01138.

35. Nelson HD, Vesco KK, Haney E, et al. Nonhormonal therapies for menopausal hot flashes: Systematic review and meta-analysis. JAMA. 2006;295:2057–71.

36. Capriglione S, Plotti F, Montera R, et al. Role of paroxetine in the management of hot flashes in gynecological cancer survivors: Results of the first randomized single-center controlled trial. Gynecol Oncol. 2016;143:584–88.

37. Carroll DG, Kelley KW. Use of antidepressants for management of hot flashes. Pharmacotherapy. 2009;29:1357–74.

38. A. Pollack, "F.D.A. Panel Advises Against Two Medicines to Treat Hot Flashes," *New York Times,* March 4, 2013.

39. http://www.independent.ie/life/health-wellbeing/health-features/the-menopause-everything-you-need-to-know-about-the-change-35837358.html.

40. Tice JA, Ettinger B, Ensrud K, et al. Phytoestrogen supplements for the treatment of hot flashes: The Isoflavone Clover Extract Study: A randomized controlled trial. JAMA. 2003;290:207–14.

41. Grady D. Management of menopausal symptoms. N Engl J Med. 2006;355:2338–47.

42. Nelson HD, Vesco KK, Haney E, et al. Nonhormonal therapies for menopausal hot flashes: Systematic review and meta-analysis. JAMA. 2006;295:2057–71.

43. Newton KM, Reed SD, LaCroix AZ, et al. Treatment of vasomotor symptoms of menopause with black cohosh, multi-botanicals, soy, hormone therapy, or placebo. Ann Int Med. 2006;145:869–79.

Mangione C. A randomized trial of alternative medicines for vasomotor symptoms of menopause. Ann Int Med. 2006;145: 924–25.

44. Pockaj BA, Gallagher JG, Loprinzi CL, et al. Phase III double-blind, randomized, placebo-controlled crossover trial of black cohosh in the management of hot flashes: NCCTG trial N01CC. J Clin Oncol. 2006;18:2836–41.

45. Deng G, Vickers A, Yeung S, et al. Randomized, controlled trial of acupuncture for the treatment of hot flashes in breast cancer patients. J Clin Oncol. 2007;35:5584–90.

46. Herbal medicines for menopausal symptoms. Drug Ther Bull. 2009;47:2–6.

47. E. Schwartz, K. Holtorf, and D. Brownstein, "The Truth About Hormone Therapy," *Wall Street Journal,* March 16, 2009; http://online.wsj.com/article/SB123717056802137143.html#mod =todays_us_opinion.

48. Brinton RD, Proffitt P, Tran J, Luu R. Equilin, a principal component of the estrogen replacement therapy Premarin, increases the growth of cortical neurons via an NMDA receptor-dependent mechanism. Exp Neurol. 1997;147:211–20.

49. Santoro N, Braunstein GD, Butts CL. Compounded bioidentical hormones in endocrinology practice: An Endocrine Society scientific statement. J Clin Endocrinol Metab. 2016;101:1318–43.

50. Thompson JJ, Ritenbaugh C, Richter M. Why women choose compounded bioidentical hormone therapy: Lessons from a qualitative study of menopause decision-making. BMC Women's Health. 2017;17:97.

51. Rosenthal MS. The Wiley Protocol: An analysis of ethical issues. Menopause. 2008;15:1014–22.

52. Quoted in Smyth, "Women Told Hormone Replacement Therapy."

Chapter 3: Matters of the Heart

1. Siegel RL, Miller KD, Jemal A. Cancer statistics, CA Cancer J Clin. 2018;68:7–30.

2. Assessing the odds. Lancet. 1997;350:1563.

3. Gulati M, Shaw LJ, Merz CNB. Myocardial ischemia in women—lessons from the NHLBI WISE study. Clin Cardiol. 2012;35:141–48.

4. M. Legato and C. Colman, *The Female Heart: The Truth About Women and Heart Disease* (New York: Perennial Currents, 2000). See also N. Goldberg, *Women Are Not Small Men: Life-Saving Strategies for Preventing and Healing Heart Disease in Women* (New York: Ballantine, 2003).

5. Sinaceur M, Heath C, Cole S. Emotional and deliberative reactions to a public crisis: Mad cow disease in France. Psychol Sci. 2005;16:247–54.

6. Patnaik JL, Byers T, Diguiseppe C, et al. Cardiovascular disease competes with breast cancer as the leading cause of death for older females diagnosed with breast cancer: A retrospective cohort study. Breast Can Res. 2011;13:R64.

7. Quoted in Goodman A, Helwick C. New data on prognostic factors, disease detection, drug toxicities, and treatment adherence presented at SABCS. ASCO Post, February 25, 2017, 18.

8. Mehta LS, Watson KE, Barac C, et al. Cardiovascular disease and breast cancer: Where these entities intersect. A scientific statement from the American Heart Association. Circulation. 2018;137; doi.org/10.1161/CIR.0000000000000556.

9. Colditz GA, Willett WC, Stampfer MJ, et al. Menopause and the risk of coronary heart disease in women. N Engl J Med. 1987;316: 1105–10.

Stampfer MJ, Colditz GA. Estrogen replacement therapy and coronary heart disease: A quantitative assessment of the epidemiologic evidence. Prev Med. 1991;20:47–63.

10. Barrett-Connor E, Bush TL. Estrogen and coronary heart disease in women. JAMA. 1991;265:1861–67. See also Barrett-Connor E, Grady D. Hormone replacement therapy, heart disease, and other considerations. Annu Rev Public Health. 1998;19:55–72.

11. Goldman L, Tosteson AN. Uncertainty about postmenopausal estrogen: Time for action, not debate. N Engl J Med. 1991;325:800–802.

12. Grodstein F, Manson JE, Colditz GA, et al. A prospective observational study of postmenopausal hormone therapy and primary prevention of cardiovascular disease. Ann Intern Med. 2000;133:933–41.

13. Jacobson BK, Knutson SF, Fraser GE. Age at natural menopause and total mortality and mortality from ischemic heart disease: The Adventist Health Study. J Clin Epidemiol. 1999;52:303–7.

Rivera CM, Grossardt BR, Rhodes DJ, et al. Increased cardiovascular mortality after early bilateral oophorectomy. Menopause. 2009;16:15–23.

14. Chalmers TC, Celano P, Sacks HS, Smith H Jr. Bias in treatment assignment in controlled clinical trials. N Engl J Med. 1983;309:1358–61.

Sacks H, Chalmers TC, Smith H Jr. Randomized versus historical controls for clinical trials. Am J Med. 1982;72:233–40.

Colditz GA, Miller JN, Mosteller F. How study design affects outcomes in comparisons of therapy. I. Medical. Stat Med. 1989;8:441–54.

15. D. L. Sackett et al., *Evidence-Based Medicine: How to Practice and Teach EBM* (New York: Churchill Livingstone, 1997).

16. Concato J, Shah N, Horwitz RI. Randomized, controlled trials, observational studies, and the hierarchy of research designs. N Engl J Med. 2000;342:1887–92.

Steen RG, Dager SR. Evaluating the evidence for evidence-based medicine: Are randomized clinical trials less flawed than other forms of peer-reviewed medical research? FASEB J. 2013;27: 3430–36.

Hellman S. Of mice but not men. Problems of the randomized clinical trial. N Engl J Med. 1991;324:1585–89.

17. Benson K, Hartz AJ. A comparison of observational studies and randomized, controlled trials. N Engl J Med. 2000;342:1878–86.

18. Poynard T, Munteanu M, Ratziu V, et al. Truth survival in clinical research: An evidence-based requiem? Ann Intern Med. 2002;136: 888–95.

19. D. Healy, *Pharmageddon* (Berkeley: University of California Press, 2012), 95.

20. Rossouw JE, Anderson GL, Prentice RL, et al. Risks and benefits of estrogen plus progestin in healthy postmenopausal women: Principal results from the Women's Health Initiative Randomized Controlled Trial. JAMA. 2002;288:321–33.

21. Speroff L. A clinician's review of the WHI-related literature. Int J Fertil. 2004;49:252–67.

22. Rossouw JE, Prentice RI, Manson JE, et al. Postmenopausal hormone therapy and risk of cardiovascular disease by age and years since menopause. JAMA. 2007;297:1465–77.

23. Grodstein F, Manson JE, Stampfer MJ. Hormone therapy and coronary heart disease: The role of time since menopause and age at hormone initiation. J Women's Health. 2006;15:35–44.

24. Salpeter SR, Walsh JM, Greyber E, et al. Brief report: Coronary heart disease events associated with hormone therapy in younger and older women. A meta-analysis. J Gen Intern Med. 2006;21: 363–66.

25. Schierbeck LL, Rejnmark L, Landbo C, et al. Effect of hormone replacement therapy on cardiovascular events and recently postmenopausal women: Randomized trial. BMJ. 2012;345:e6409.

26. Shapiro S. Risks of estrogen plus progestin therapy: A sensitivity analysis of the findings in the Women's Health Initiative randomized controlled trial. Climacteric. 2003;6:302–10.

27. Bhavnani BR, Strickler RC. Menopausal hormone therapy. J Obstet Gynaecol Can. 2005;27:137–62.

28. C. Dean, *Making Sense of Science* (Cambridge, MA: Belknap Press, 2017), 234.

29. Hulley S, Grady D, Bush T, et al. Randomized trial of estrogen plus progestin for secondary prevention of coronary heart disease in postmenopausal women. JAMA. 1998;280:605–13.

30. Mikkola TS, Clarkson TB. Estrogen replacement therapy, atherosclerosis, and vascular function. Cardiovasc Res. 2002;53:605–19.

31. Herrington DM, Reboussin DM, Brosnihan KB, et al. Effects of estrogen replacement on the progression of coronary artery atherosclerosis. N Engl J Med. 2000;343:522–29.

    Hodis HN, Mack WJ, Lobo RA, et al. Estrogen in the prevention of atherosclerosis. Ann Intern Med. 2001;135:939–53.

    Hodis HN, Collins P, Mack WJ. The timing hypothesis for coronary heart disease prevention with hormone therapy: Past, present and future perspective. Climacteric. 2012;15:217–28.

32. Hodis HN, Mack WJ, Henderson VW, et al. Vascular effects of early versus late postmenopausal treatment with estradiol. N Engl J Med. 2016;374:1221–31.

33. Sprague BL, Trentham-Dietz A, Cronin KA. A sustained decline in postmenopausal hormone use: Results from the National Health and Nutrition Examination Survey, 1999–2010. Obstet Gynecol. 2012;120:595–603.

34. Mikkola TS, Tuomikoski P, Lyytinen H, et al. Increased cardiovascular mortality risk in women discontinuing postmenopausal hormone therapy. J Clin Endocrinol Metab. 2015;100:4588–94.

    Tuomikoski P, Lyytinen H, Korhonen P, et al. Coronary heart

disease mortality and hormone therapy before and after the Women's Health Initiative. Obstet Gynecol. 2014;124:947–53.

35. T. Parker-Pope, "How NIH Misread Hormonal Study in 2002," *Wall Street Journal,* July 9, 2007.

36. T. Parker-Pope, "Palpitations over a New Pill for Kids," *New York Times,* July 13, 2008; http://www.nytimes.com/2008/07/13/week inreview/13parker.html.

37. Olotu BS, Shepherd MD, Novak S, et al. Use of statins and the risk of incident diabetes: A retrospective cohort study. Am J Cardiovasc Drugs. 2016;16:377–90.

    Sattar N, Preiss D, Murray HM, et al. Statins and risk of incident diabetes: A collaborative meta-analysis of randomised statin trials. Lancet. 2010;375:735–42.

38. B. H. Roberts, *The Truth About Statins: Risks and Alternatives to Cholesterol-Lowering Drugs* (New York: Pocket Books, 2012). See also H. Rosenberg and D. Allard, "Evidence for Caution: Women and statin use," 2007. Women and Health Protection report, Canada. http://www.whpapsf.ca/pdf/statinEvidenceCaution.pdf.

39. Walsh JME, Pignone M. Drug treatment of hyperlipidemia in women. JAMA. 2004;291:2243–52.

40. For an excellent history of how Ancel Keys invented and promoted cholesterol as being a major culprit in heart disease and how the American Heart Association supported that belief in the virtual absence of supporting evidence, see G. Taubes, *The Case Against Sugar* (New York: Knopf, 2016).

41. Kannel WB, Hjortland MC, McNamara PM, et al. Menopause and risk of cardiovascular disease: The Framingham study. Ann Intern Med. 1976;85:447–52.

42. Krumholz HM, Seeman TE, Merrill SS, et al. Lack of association between cholesterol and coronary heart disease mortality and morbidity and all-cause mortality in persons older than 70 years. JAMA. 1994;272:1335–40.

43. G. Taubes, *Good Calories, Bad Calories* (New York: Random House, 2007).

44. Dehghan M, Mente A, Zhang X, et al. Associations of fats and carbohydrate intake with cardiovascular disease and mortality in 18 countries from five continents (PURE): A prospective cohort study. Lancet. 2017; DOI: 10.1016/S0140-6736(17)32252-3.

    Another huge study—a meta-analysis of cohort studies of nearly 350,000 participants who were followed for five to twenty-three years—showed that "intake of saturated fat was not associated with an increased risk of CHD, stroke, or CVD.... Consideration of age, sex, and study quality did not change the results." Siri-Tarino PW, Sun Q, Hu FB, Krauss RM. Meta-analysis of prospective cohort studies evaluating the association of saturated fat with cardiovascular disease. Am J Clin Nutr. 2010;91: 535–46.

45. Howard Hodis, interviewed by Cynthia Fox for *Bioscience Technology,* March 16, 2015.

    Hodis HN, Mack WJ, Henderson VW, et al. Vascular effects of early versus late postmenopausal treatment with estradiol. N Engl J Med. 2016;374:1221–31.

46. Hodis HN, Collins P, Mack WJ, Schierbeck LL. The timing hypothesis for coronary heart disease prevention with hormone therapy: Past, present and future in perspective. Climacteric. 2012;15:217–28.

47. Gorsky RD, Koplan JP, Peterson HB, et al. Relative risks and benefits of long-term estrogen replacement therapy: A decision analysis. Obstet Gynecol. 1994;83:161–66.

48. Col NF, Eckman MH, Karas RH, et al. Patient-specific decisions about hormone replacement therapy in postmenopausal women. JAMA. 1997;277:1140–47.

49. Arnson Y, et al. Hormone replacement therapy associated with lower mortality. Press release from the American College of

Cardiology, March 8, 2017; https://www.eurekalert.org/pub_releases
/2017-03/acoc-hrt030617.php.

Chapter 4: Breaking Bad

1. Alswat KA. Gender disparities in osteoporosis. J Clin Med Res. 2017;9:382–87.
2. Cummings SR, Melton LJ. Epidemiology and outcomes of osteoporotic fractures. Lancet. 2002;359:1761–67.
3. Cummings SR, Nevitt MC, Browner WS, et al. Risk factors for hip fracture in white women. N Engl J Med. 1995;332:767–74.
4. Brauer CA, Coca-Perraillon M, Cutler DM, Rosen AB. Incidence and mortality of hip fractures in the United States. JAMA. 2009;302:1573–79.

   Goldacre MJ, Roberts SE, Yeates D. Mortality after admission to hospital with fractured neck of femur: Database study. BMJ. 2002;325:868–69.
5. Vestergaard P, Rejnmark L, Mosekilde L. Increased mortality in patients with a hip fracture—effect of pre-morbid conditions in post-fracture complications. Osteoporos Int. 2007;18:1583–93.

   Vestergaard P, Rejnmark L, Mosekilde L. Loss of life years after a hip fracture: Effects of age and sex. Acta Orthopaedica. 2009;80: 525–30.
6. Empana JP, Dargent-Molina P, Béart G, et al. Effect of hip fracture on mortality in elderly women: The EPIDOS prospective study. J Am Geriatr Soc. 2004;52:685–90. The absolute numbers were 112 deaths per 1,000 woman-years in the hip-fracture group compared with 27.3 deaths per 1,000 woman-years for the 6,115 women who did not have any fractures.
7. Von Friesendorff M, McGuigan FE, Wizert A, et al. Hip fracture, mortality risk, and cause of death over two decades. Osteoporos Int. 2016;27:2945–53.
8. Wilson JF. New treatments for growing scourge of brittle bones. Ann Intern Med. 2004;140:153–56.

9. Seeman E, Delmas PD. Bone quality—the material and structural basis of bone strength and fragility. N Engl J Med. 2006; 354:2250–61.

10. Albright F, Bloomberg E, Smith PH. Post-menopausal osteoporosis. Trans Assoc Am Physicians. 1940;55:298–305.

   Albright F, Burnett CH, et al. Osteomalacia and late rickets: the various etiologies met in the United States with emphasis on that resulting from a specific form of renal acidosis, the therapeutic indications for each etiological sub-group, and the relationship between osteomalacia and Milkman's syndrome. Medicine. 1946;25:399–479.

   Gordan GS. Estrogen and postmenopausal osteoporosis. Ann Intern Med. 1993;118:155.

   Henneman PH, Wallach S. A review of the prolonged use of estrogens and androgens in postmenopausal and senile osteoporosis. AMA Arch Intern Med. 1957;100:715–23.

11. Zhao J-G, Zeng X-T, Wang J, Liu L. Association between calcium or vitamin D supplementation and fracture incidence in community-dwelling older adults: A systematic review and meta-analysis. JAMA. 2017;318:2466–82.

12. Bischoff-Ferrari HA, Dawson-Hughes B, Baron JA, et al. Calcium intake and hip fracture risk in men and women: A meta-analysis of prospective cohort studies and randomized controlled trials. Am J Clin Nutr. 2007;86:1780–90.

13. Jackson RD, LaCroix AZ, Gass M, et al. Calcium plus vitamin D supplementation and the risk of fractures. N Engl J Med. 2006;354:669–83.

14. Nachtigall LE, Nachtigall RH, Nachtigall RD, et al. Estrogen replacement. I. A 10-year prospective study in the relationship to osteoporosis. Obstet Gynecol. 1979;53:277–81.

   Christiansen C, Christiansen MA, Transol I. Bone mass in postmenopausal women after withdrawal of oestrogen/progestogen replacement therapy. Lancet. 1981;1:459–61.

Lobo RA, McCormick W, Singer F, et al. Depomedroxyprogesterone acetate compared with conjugated estrogens for the treatment of postmenopausal women. Obstet Gynecol. 1984;63: 1–5.

15. Peck WA, Barrett-Connor E, Buckwalter JA, et al. Consensus conference: Osteoporosis. JAMA. 1984;252:799–802.

Consensus Development Conference: Prophylaxis and treatment of osteoporosis. BMJ. 1987;295:914–15.

16. Weiss NS, Ure CL, Ballard JH, et al. Decreased risk of fractures of the hip and lower forearm with postmenopausal use of estrogen. N Engl J Med. 1980;303:1195–98.

Kiel DP, Felson DT, Anderson JJ, et al. Hip fracture and the use of estrogens in postmenopausal women: The Framingham study. N Engl J Med. 1987;317:1169–74.

17. Naessén T, Persson I, Adami HO, et al. Hormone replacement therapy and the risk for first hip fracture. A prospective, population-based cohort study. Ann Intern Med. 1990;113:95–103.

Michaëlsson K, Baron JA, Farahmand BY, et al. Hormone replacement therapy and risk of hip fracture: Population-based case-controlled study. BMJ. 1998;316:1858–63.

Von Friesendorff M, McGuigan FE, Wizert A, et al. Hip fracture, mortality risk, and cause of death over two decades. Osteoporos Int. 2016;27:2945–53.

18. Rossouw JE, Anderson GL, Prentice RL, et al. Risks and benefits of estrogen plus progestin in healthy postmenopausal women: Principal results from the Women's Health Initiative Randomized Controlled Trial. JAMA. 2002;288:321–33.

Cauley JA, Robbins J, Chen Z, et al. Effects of estrogen plus progestin on risk of fracture and bone mineral density: The Women's Health Initiative Randomized Trial. JAMA. 2003;290:1929–38.

Manson JE, Chlebowski RT, Stefanick ML, et al. The Women's Health Initiative Hormone Therapy Trials: Update and overview of health outcomes during the intervention and post-stopping phases. JAMA. 2013;310:1353–68.

19. Col, NF, Bowlby LA, McGarry K. The role of menopausal hormone therapy in preventing osteoporotic fractures: A critical review of the clinical evidence. Minerva Med. 2005;96:331–42.

20. Lindsay R, Hart DM, MacLean A, et al. Bone response to termination of oestrogen treatment. Lancet. 1978;1:1325–27.

21. Grady D, Rubin SM, Petitti DB, et al. Hormone therapy to prevent disease and prolong life in postmenopausal women. Ann Intern Med. 1992;117:1016–37.

22. Ettinger B, Grady D. The waning effect of postmenopausal estrogen therapy on osteoporosis. N Engl J Med. 1993;329:1192–93.

23. https://www.mayoclinic.org/diseases-conditions/osteoporosis /diagnosis-treatment/drc-20351974.

24. G. N. Grob, *Aging Bones: A Short History of Osteoporosis* (Baltimore: Johns Hopkins University Press, 2014), xv.

25. T. Parker-Pope, *The Hormone Decision* (Emmaus, PA: Rodale, 2007).

26. Chestnut CH. Theoretical overview: Bone development, peak bone mass, bone loss, and fracture risk. Am J Med. 1991;91:2S–4S.

    Eisman JA, Sambrook PN, Kelly PJ, et al. Exercise and its interaction with genetic influences in the determination of bone mineral density. Am J Med. 1991;91:5S–9S.

27. Riggs BL, Hodgson SF, O'Fallon WM, et al. Effect of fluoride treatment on the fracture rate in postmenopausal women with osteoporosis. N Engl J Med. 1990;322:802–9.

    Heaney RP. Bone mass, bone fragility, and the decision to treat. JAMA. 1998;280:2119–20.

    Heaney RP, Recker RR. Combination and sequential therapy for osteoporosis. N Engl J Med. 2005;353:624–25.

28. For example, John A. Kanis, a leading British authority, noted that all definitions of *osteoporosis* based on bone density were arbitrary

and that other factors contributed to bone fragility. Kanis JA. Osteoporosis and osteopenia. J Bone Miner Res. 1990;5:209–10.

29. Ettinger B, Miller P, McClung MR. Use of bone densitometry results for decisions about therapy for osteoporosis. Ann Int Med. 1996;125:623.

30. Grob, *Aging Bones*. See also Grob G. From aging to pathology: The case of osteoporosis. J Hist Med Allied Sci. 2010:1–39.

31. Ettinger B, Miller P, McClung MR. Use of bone densitometry results for decisions about therapy for osteoporosis. Ann Int Med. 1996;125:623.

32. Cheung AM, Detsky AS. Osteoporosis and fractures. Missing the bridge? JAMA. 2008;299:1468–70.

33. Judy Foreman, "Should Bone Loss Always Be Treated?," *Los Angeles Times,* June 13, 2005.

34. G. N. Grob and A. V. Horwitz, *Diagnosis, Therapy, and Evidence: Conundrums in Modern American Medicine* (New Brunswick, NJ: Rutgers University Press, 2010), 195.

35. Tella SH, Gallagher JC. Prevention and treatment of postmenopausal osteoporosis. J Steroid Biochem Mol Biol. 2014;142: 155–70.

36. Wang Z, Ward MM, Chan L, Bhattacharyya T. Adherence to oral bisphosphonates and the risk of subtrochanteric and femoral shaft fractures among female Medicare beneficiaries. Osteoporos Int. 2014;25:2109–16.

37. Odvina C, Zerwekh J, Rao D, et al. Severely suppressed bone turnover: A potential complication of alendronate therapy. J Clin Endocrinol Metab. 2005;90:1294–1301.

Saita Y, Ishijima M, Kaneko K. Atypical femoral fractures and bisphosphonate use: Current evidence and clinical implications. Ther Adv Chron Dis. 2015;6:185–93.

Kharwadkar N, Mayne B, Lawrence JE, et al. Bisphosphonates and atypical subtrochanteric fractures of the femur. Bone Joint Res. 2017;6:144–53.

Schilcher J, Koeppen V, Aspenberg P. Risk of atypical femoral fracture during and after bisphosphonate use. N Engl J Med. 2014;371:974–76.

Shane E, Burr D, Abrahamsen B, et al. Atypical subtrochanteric and diaphyseal femoral fractures: Second report of a task force of the American Society for Bone and Mineral Research. J Bone Miner Res. 2014;29:1–23.

Meier RPH, Perneger TV, Stern R, et al. Increasing occurrence of atypical femoral fractures associated with bisphosphonate use. Arch Intern Med. 2012;172:930–36.

38. Drieling RL, LaCroix AZ, Beresford SAA, et al. Long-term oral bisphosphonate therapy and fractures in older women: The Women's Health Initiative. J Am Geriatr Soc. 2017;65:1924–31.

39. Langer RD, Simon JA, Pines A, et al. Menopausal hormone therapy for primary prevention: Why the USPSTF is wrong. Climacteric. 2017;20:402–13.

40. Ettinger B, Black DM, Mitlak BH, et al. Reduction of vertebral fracture risk in postmenopausal women with osteoporosis treated with raloxifene: Results from a three-year randomized clinical trial. JAMA. 1999;282:637–45; erratum JAMA. 1999;282:2124.

Grady D, Ettinger B, Moscarelli E, et al. Multiple outcomes of raloxifene evaluation investigators. Safety and adverse effects associated with raloxifene: Multiple outcomes of raloxifene evaluation. Obstet Gynecol. 2004;104:837–44.

Gambacciani M, Levancini M. Hormone replacement therapy and the prevention of postmenopausal osteoporosis. Prz Menopauzalny. 2014;13:213–20.

41. Silverman SL. Calcitonin. Endocrinol Metab Clin North Amer. 2003;32:273–84.

Watts NB, Worley K, Solis A, et al. Comparison of risedronate to alendronate and calcitonin for early reduction of nonvertebral fracture risk: Results from a managed care administrative claims database. J Manag Care Pharm. 2004;10:142–51.

Kung AW, Pasion EG, Sofiyan M, et al. A comparison of teriparatide and calcitonin therapy in postmenopausal Asian women with osteoporosis: A 6-month study. Curr Med Res Opin. 2006;22:929–37.

42. Eriksen DR, Keaveny TM, Gallagher ER, et al. Literature review: The effects of teriparatide therapy at the hip in patients with osteoporosis. Bone. 2014;67:246–56.

43. Miller PD, Hattersley G, Riis BJ, et al. Effect of abaloparatide vs. placebo on new vertebral fractures in postmenopausal women with osteoporosis: A randomized clinical trial. JAMA. 2016;316: 722–33.

44. Qi W-X, Lin F, He A-N. Incidence and risk of denosumab-related hypocalcemia in cancer patients: A systematic review and pooled analysis of randomized controlled studies. Curr Med Res Opin. 2013;29:1067–73.

45. Saag KG, Peterson J, Brandi ML, et al. Romosozumab or alendronate for fracture prevention in women with osteoporosis. N Engl J Med. 2017;377:1417–27.

Rosen CJ. Romosozumab — promising or practice changing? N Engl J Med. 2017;377:1479–80.

46. http://www.fiercebiotech.com/biotech/safety-scare-prompts -fda-to-reject-amgen-s-romosozumab.

Chapter 5: Losing and Using Our Minds

1. K. Fackelmann, "Forever Smart: Does Estrogen Enhance Memory?," *Science News* 147 (1995): 74–75.

2. Alzheimer's Association, 2014 Alzheimer's Disease Facts and Figures, https://www.alz.org/documents_custom/2014_facts_and_figures _release.pdf.

3. Alzheimer's Association. 2017 Alzheimer's disease facts and figures. Alzheimer's Dement 2017;13:325–73. The sixty-six-seconds number is calculated by dividing the number of seconds in a year

(31,536,000) by the number of new cases in a year (479,900), which comes to 65.7 seconds. Using the same method of calculation for 2050, 31,536,000 divided by 959,000 is 32.8 seconds. Data based on Hebert LE, Weuve J, Scherr PA, Evans DA. Alzheimer disease in the United States (2010–2050) estimated using the 2010 Census. Neurol. 2013;80:1778–83.

4. Hebert LE, Weuve J, Scherr PA, Evans DA. Alzheimer disease in the United States (2010–2050) estimated using the 2010 Census. Neurol. 2013;80:1778–83.

5. Alzheimer's Association. 2017 Alzheimer's disease facts and figures. Alzheimer's Dement. 2017;13:325–73.

6. Ari A, Frölich L, Ballard C, et al. Effect of idalopirdine as adjunct to cholinesterase inhibitor on change in cognition in patients with Alzheimer disease: Three randomized clinical trials. JAMA. 2018;19:13–42.

   Bennett DA. Lack of benefit with idalopirdine for Alzheimer disease: Another therapeutic failure in a complex disease process. JAMA. 2018;19:123–25.

7. Here's one: Zandi PP, Carlson MC, Plassman BL, et al. Hormone replacement therapy and incidence of Alzheimer disease in older women: The Cache County Study. JAMA. 2002;288:2123–29.

8. Shumaker SA, Legault C, Rapp SR, et al. Estrogen plus progestin and the incidence of dementia and mild cognitive impairment in postmenopausal women: The Women's Health Initiative Memory Study. A randomized controlled trial. JAMA. 2003;289:2651–62.

9. Ibid., 2660.

10. Shumaker SA, Legault C, Kuller L, et al. Conjugated equine estrogens and incidence of probable dementia and mild cognitive impairment in postmenopausal women: Women's Health Initiative Memory Study. JAMA. 2004;291:2947–58.

11. Schneider LS. Estrogen and dementia: Insights from the Women's Health Initiative Memory Study. JAMA. 2004;291:3005–7.

12. Espeland MA, Rapp SR, Shumaker SA, et al. Conjugated equine estrogens and global cognitive function in postmenopausal women: Women's Health Initiative Memory Study. JAMA. 2004; 291:2959–68.

13. Ibid.

14. Speroff, L. A clinician's review of the WHI-related literature. Int J Fertil. 2004;49:252–67. Typically for the contradictory interpretations and conclusions among the many WHI investigators, one, Lon Schneider, wrote that "the risk of dementia remained when women who probably had cognitive impairment at baseline were removed." Schneider LS. Estrogen and dementia: Insights from the Women's Health Initiative Memory Study. JAMA. 2004; 291:3005–7.

15. Simpkins JW, Singh M, for the CARPE group. Consortium for the Assessment of Research on Progestins and Estrogens: Letter to the Editor. J Women's Health. 2004;13:1165–68.

    Wickelgren I. Estrogen research: Brain researchers try to salvage estrogen treatments. Science. 2003;302:1138–39.

    Simpkins JM, Singh M. More than a decade of estrogen neuroprotection. Alzheimer's Dement. 2008;4:S131–36.

16. Shumaker SA, Legault C, Rapp SR, et al. Estrogen plus progestin and the incidence of dementia and mild cognitive impairment in postmenopausal women. The Women's Health Initiative Memory Study: A randomized controlled trial. JAMA. 2003;289:2651–62.

17. Bhavnani BR, Strickler RC. Menopausal hormone therapy. J Obstet Gynaecol Can. 2005;27:137–62.

18. Espeland MA, Rapp SR, Shumaker SA, et al. Conjugated equine estrogens and global cognitive function in postmenopausal women: Women's Health Initiative Memory Study. JAMA. 2004;291:2959–68.

19. R. D. Fields, *The Other Brain: The Scientific and Medical Breakthroughs That Will Heal Our Brains and Revolutionize Our Health* (New York: Simon and Schuster, 2011).

20. Marriott LK, Wenk GL. Neurobiological consequences of long-term estrogen therapy. Curr Dir Psychol Sci. 2004;13:173–76.

21. Arevalo MA, Azcoitia I, Garcia-Segura LM. The neuroprotective actions of oestradiol and oestrogen receptors. Nat Rev Neurosci. 2015;16:17–29.

    Jones KJ. Steroid hormones and neurotrophism: Relationship to nerve injury. Metab Brain Dis. 1988;3:1–16.

    Gould E, Woolley CS, Frankfurt M, et al. Gonadal steroids regulate dendritic spine density in hippocampal pyramidal cells in adulthood. J Neurosci. 1990;10:1286–91.

    Sherwin BB. Hormones and the brain. J Obstet Gynaecol Can. 2001;23:1102–4.

22. Squire L. Memory in the hippocampus: A synthesis from findings with rats, monkeys, and humans. Psychol Rev. 1992;99:195–231.

    Shughrue PJ, Lane MV, Merchenthaler I. Comparative distribution of estrogen receptor-alpha and -beta mRNA in the rat central nervous system. J Comp Neurol. 1997;388:507–25.

    S. Alves and B. McEwen, *Estrogen and Brain Function: Implications for Aging and Dementia* (New York: Springer, 1999).

    Maki PM, Henderson VW. Hormone therapy, dementia, and cognition: The Women's Health Initiative ten years on. Climacteric. 2012;15:256–62.

23. Opendak M, Briones BA, Gould E. Social behavior, hormones and adult neurogenesis. Front Neuroendocrinol. 2016;41:71–86.

24. Gould E, Woolley CS, Frankfurt M, et al. Gonadal steroids regulate dendritic spine density in hippocampal pyramidal cells in adulthood. J Neurosci. 1990;10:1286–91.

25. Woolley CS, Wenzel HJ, Schwartzkroin PA. Estradiol increases the frequency of multiple synapse boutons in the hippocampal CA1 region of the adult female rat. J Comp Neurol. 1996;373:108–17.

    R. E. Brinton, "Biochemistry of Learning and Memory," in J. L. Martinez and R. B. Kesner, eds., *Learning and Memory: A Biological View* (San Diego: Academic Press, 1991), 199–246.

Singh M, Meyer EM, Millard WJ, Simpkin JW. Ovarian steroid deprivation results in a reversal learning impairment and compromised cholinergic function in female Sprague Dawley rats. Brain Res. 1994;644:305–12.

Simpkins JW, Green PS, Gridley KE, et al. Role of estrogen replacement therapy and memory enhancement and the prevention of neuronal loss associated with Alzheimer's disease. Am J Med. 1997;103:19S–25S.

Wise P, Smith M, Dubal D, et al. Neuroendocrine influences and repercussions of the menopause. Endocr Rev. 1999;20:243–48.

Zhao L, Mao Z, Chen S, et al. Early Intervention with an estrogen receptor β-selective phytoestrogenic formulation prolongs survival, improves spatial recognition memory, and slows progression of amyloid pathology in a female mouse model of Alzheimer's disease. J Alzheimer's Dis. 2013;37:403–19.

26. Brinton RD. 17 beta estradiol induction of filopodial growth and cultured hippocampal neurons within minutes of exposure. Mol Cell Neurosci. 1993;4:36–46.

Brinton RD. Estrogen-induced plasticity from cells to circuits: Predictions for cognitive function. Trends Pharmacol. 2009;30:212–22.

McEwen B, Alves S. Estrogen actions in the central nervous system. Endocr Rev. 1999;20:279–307.

27. Bartus RT, Dean RL, Beer B, Lippa AS. The cholinergic hypothesis of memory dysfunction. Science. 1982;217:408–17.

Luine VN. Estradiol increases choline acetyltransferase activity in specific basal forebrain nuclei and projection areas of female rats. Exp Neurol. 1985;89:484–90.

28. Brinton RD, Proffitt P, Tran J, Luu R. Equilin, a principal component of the estrogen replacement therapy Premarin, increases the growth of cortical neurons via an NMDA receptor-dependent mechanism. Exp Neurol. 1997;147:211–20.

Brinton RD. Estrogen-induced plasticity from cells to circuits: Predictions for cognitive function. Trends Pharmacol. 2009;30: 212–22.

Bhavnani BR, Strickler RC. Menopausal hormone therapy. J Obstet Gynaecol Can. 2005;27:137–62.

Gupta PB, Kuperwasser C. Contributions of estrogen to ER-negative breast tumor growth. J Steroid Biochem Mol Biol. 2006; 102:71–78.

29. Brinton RD, Chen S, Montoya M, et al. The Women's Health Initiative estrogen replacement therapy is neurotrophic and neuro-protective. Neurobiol of Aging. 2000;21:475–96.

Horsburgh K, Mhairi Macrae I, Carswell H. Estrogen is neu-roprotective via an apolipoprotein E-dependent mechanism in a mouse model of global ischemia. J Cereb Blood Flow Metab. 2002;22:1189–95.

Nilsen J, Brinton R. Mechanism of estrogen-mediated neuropro-tection: Regulation of mitochondrial calcium and Bcl-2 expression. Proc Natl Acad Sci USA. 2003;100:2842–47.

30. Toran-Allerand CD. The estrogen/neurotrophin connection during neural development: Is co-localization of estrogen receptors with the neurotrophins and their receptors biologically relevant? Dev Neurosci. 1996;18:36–48.

31. Xu H, Gouras GK, Greenfield JP, et al. Estrogen reduces neuronal generation of Alzheimer beta-amyloid peptides. Nat Med. 1998; 4:447–51.

McEwen B, Alves S. Estrogen actions in the central nervous system. Endocr Rev. 1999;20:279–307.

Brinton RD. Investigative models for determining hormone therapy–induced outcomes in brain: Evidence in support of a healthy cell bias of estrogen action. Ann NY Acad Sci. 2005;1052:57–74.

32. Alvarez-de-la-Rosa M, Silva I, Nilsen J, et al. Estradiol prevents neural tau hyperphosphorylation characteristic of Alzheimer's dis-ease. Ann NY Acad Sci. 2005;1052:210–24.

33. Dhandapani KM, Brann DW. Estrogen-astrocyte interactions: Implications for neuroprotection. BMC Neurosci. 2002;3:6.

Arevalo MA, Azcoitia I, Garcia-Segura LM. The neuroprotective actions of oestradiol and oestrogen receptors. Nat Rev Neurosci. 2015;16:17–29.

Norbury R, Cutter WJ, Compton J, et al. The neuroprotective effects of estrogen on the aging brain. Exp Gerontol. 2003;38: 109–17.

34. Sherwin BB. Hormones and the brain. J Obstet Gynaecol Can. 2001;23:1102–4.

Sherwin BB. Estrogen and cognitive functioning in women: Lessons we have learned. Behav Neurosci. 2012;126:123–27.

35. Greene RA. Estrogen and cerebral blood flow: A mechanism to explain the impact of estrogen on the incidence and treatment of Alzheimer's disease. Int J Fertil Women's Med. 2000;45:253–57.

36. Brinton RD. Estrogen-induced plasticity from cells to circuits: Predictions for cognitive function. Trends Pharmacol. 2009;30: 212–22.

37. Resnick SM, Henderson VW. Hormone therapy and risk of Alzheimer's disease: A critical time. JAMA. 2002;288:2170–72.

Resnick SM, Maki PM, Rapp SR, et al. Effects of combination estrogen plus progestin hormone treatment on cognition and affect. J Clin Endocrinol Metab. 2006;91:1802–10.

38. S. Carpenter, "Does Estrogen Protect Memory?," *American Psychological Association Monitor* (January 2001): 52.

39. Caldwell BM, Watson RI. An evaluation of psychological effects of sex hormone administration in aged women: Results of therapy after six months. J Gerontol. 1952;7:228–44.

40. Kantor HI, Michael CM, Shore H. Estrogen for older women. Am J Obstet Gynecol. 1973;116:115–18.

41. Sherwin BB. Estrogen and/or androgen replacement therapy and cognitive functioning in surgically menopausal women. Psychoneuroendocrinol. 1988;13:345–57.

42. B. Chester, "Restoring Remembering: Hormones and Memory," *McGill Reporter,* February 8, 2001; https://www.mcgill.ca/reporter/33/10/sherwin/.

43. Phillips SM, Sherwin BB. Effects of estrogen on memory function in surgically menopausal women. Psychoneuroendocrinol. 1992; 17:485–95.

44. Sherwin BB, Tulandi T. "Add-back" estrogen reverses cognitive deficits induced by a gonadotropin-releasing hormone agonist in women with leiomyomata uteri. J Clin Endocrinol Metab. 1996; 81:2545–49.

    Kampen DL, Sherwin BB. Estrogen use and verbal memory in healthy postmenopausal women. Obstet Gynecol. 1994;83:979–83.

    Kimura D. Estrogen replacement therapy may protect against intellectual decline in postmenopausal women. Horm Behav. 1995;29:312–21.

45. Henderson VW, Benke KS, Green RC, et al. Postmenopausal hormone therapy and Alzheimer's disease risk: Interaction with age. J Neurol Neurosurg Psychiatry. 2005;76:103–5.

46. Tang MX, Jacobs D, Stern Y, et al. Effect of oestrogen during menopause on risk and age at onset of Alzheimer's disease. Lancet. 1996;348:429–32.

47. Paganini-Hill A, Henderson VW. Estrogen replacement therapy and risk of Alzheimer disease. Arch Intern Med. 1996;156:2213–17.

48. Baldereschi M, DiCarlo A, Lepore V, et al. Estrogen replacement therapy and Alzheimer's disease in the Italian Longitudinal Study on Aging. Neurol. 1998;50:996–1002.

49. Bagger YZ, Tanko LB, Alexandersen P, et al. for the PERF Study Group. Early postmenopausal hormone therapy may prevent cognitive impairment later in life. Menopause. 2005;12:12–17.

50. Hogervorst E, Williams J, Budge M, et al. The nature of the effect of female gonadal hormone replacement therapy on cognitive function in post-menopausal women: A meta-analysis. Neurosci. 2000;101:485–512.

LeBlanc ES, Janowsky J, Chan BKS, Nelson HD. Hormone replacement therapy and cognition: Systemic review and meta-analysis. JAMA. 2001;285:1489–99.

Maki PM, Dennerstein L, Clark M, et al. Perimenopausal use of hormone therapy is associated with enhanced memory and hippocampal function later in life. Brain Res. 2011;1379:232–43.

51. Paganini-Hill A, Ross RK, Henderson BE. Postmenopausal oestrogen treatment and stroke: A prospective study. BMJ. 1988;297:519–22.

Hunt K, Vessey M, McPherson K. Mortality in a cohort of long-term users of hormone replacement therapy: An updated analysis. Br J Obstet Gynaecol. 1990;97:1080–86.

Finucane FF, Madans JH, Bush TL, et al. Decreased risk of stroke among postmenopausal hormone users: Results from a national cohort. Arch Intern Med. 1993;153:73–79.

Falkeborn M, Persson I, Terent A, et al. Hormone replacement therapy and the risk of stroke: Follow-up of a population-based cohort in Sweden. Arch Intern Med. 1993;153:1201–9.

52. Boysen G, Nyboe J, Appleyard M, et al. Stroke incidence and risk factors for stroke in Copenhagen, Denmark. Stroke. 1988;19:1345–53.

Pedersen AT, Lidegaard O, Kreiner S, et al. Hormone replacement therapy and risk of non-fatal stroke. Lancet. 1997;350:1277–83.

Petitti DB, Sidney S, Quesenberry CP Jr, et al. Ischemic stroke and use of estrogen and estrogen/progestogen as hormone replacement therapy. Stroke. 1998;29:23–28.

53. Wilson PW, Garrison RJ, Castelli WP. Postmenopausal estrogen use, cigarette smoking, and cardiovascular morbidity in women over 50: The Framingham study. N Engl J Med. 1985;313:1038–43.

Lemaitre RN, Heckbert SR, Psaty BM, et al. Hormone replacement therapy and associated risk of stroke in postmenopausal women. Arch Intern Med. 2002;162:1954–60.

54. Simon JA, Hsia J, Cauley JA, et al. Postmenopausal hormone therapy and risk of stroke: The Heart and Estrogen/Progestin Replacement Study (HERS). Circulation. 2001;103:638–42.
55. Viscoli CM, Brass LM, Kernan WN, et al. A clinical trial of estrogen replacement therapy after ischemic stroke. N Engl J Med. 2001;345:1243–49.
56. Anderson GL, Limacher M, Assaf AR, et al. Effects of conjugated equine estrogen in postmenopausal women with hysterectomy: The Women's Health Initiative Randomized Controlled Trial. JAMA. 2004;291:1701–12.
57. Maclaren K, Stevenson JC. Primary prevention of cardiovascular disease with HRT. Women's Health. 2012:8:63–74.
    Stevenson JC, Hodis HN, Pickar JH, Lobo RA. Coronary heart disease and menopause management: The swinging pendulum of HRT. Atherosclerosis. 2009;207:336–40.
58. Manson JE, Aragaki AK, Rossouw JE, et al. for the WHI Investigators. Menopausal hormone therapy and long-term all-cause and cause-specific mortality: The Women's Health Initiative Randomized Trials. JAMA. 2017;318:927–38.
59. Mastorakos G, Sakkas EG, Xydakis AM, Creatsas G. Pitfalls of the WHI's Women's Health Initiative. Ann NY Acad Sci. 2006; 1092:331–40.
60. Birge SJ. Hormone therapy and stroke. Clin Obstet Gynecol. 2008; 51:581–91.
61. Boardman HMP, Hartley L, Eisinga A, et al. Hormone therapy for preventing cardiovascular disease in post-menopausal women. Cochrane Database of Systematic Reviews. 2015;3:CD002229. doi: 10.1002/14651858.CD002229.pub4.
62. Shao H, Breitner JC, Whitmer RA, et al. Hormone therapy and Alzheimer disease dementia: New findings from the Cache County Study. Neurol. 2012;79:1846–52. See also Whitmer RA, Quesenberry CP, Zhou J, Yaffe K. Timing of hormone therapy and dementia: The critical window theory revisited. Ann Neurol. 2011;69:163–69.

63. Brinton RD. Investigative models for determining hormone therapy–induced outcomes in brain: Evidence in support of a healthy cell bias of estrogen action. Ann NY Acad Sci. 2005; 1052:57.

64. Sherwin BB. Hormones and the brain. J Obstet Gynaecol Can. 2001;23:1103.

65. Sherwin BB. Estrogen and cognitive functioning in women: Lessons we have learned. Behav Neurosci. 2012;126:123–27.

66. Zandi PP, Carlson MC, Plassman BL, et al. Hormone replacement therapy and incidence of Alzheimer disease in older women: The Cache County Study. JAMA. 2002;288:2123–29.

    Resnick SR, Henderson VW. Hormone therapy and risk of Alzheimer's disease: A critical time. JAMA. 2002;288:2170–72.

67. Maki PM, Dennerstein L, Clark M, et al. Perimenopausal use of hormone therapy is associated with enhanced memory and hippocampal function later in life. Brain Res. 2011;1379:232–43.

    Maki PM, Henderson VW. Hormone therapy, dementia, and cognition: The Women's Health Initiative ten years on. Climacteric. 2012;15:256–62.

    Henderson VW, Benke KS, Green RC, et al. Postmenopausal hormone therapy and Alzheimer's disease risk: Interaction with age. J Neurol Neurosurg Psychiatry. 2005;76:103–5.

    Henderson VW. Alzheimer's disease: Review of hormone therapy trials and implications for treatment and prevention after menopause. J Steroid Biochem Mol Biol. 2014;142:99–106.

    MacLennan AH, Henderson VW, Paine BJ, et al. Hormone therapy, timing of initiation and cognition in women aged older than 60 years: The REMEMBER pilot study. Menopause. 2006;13: 28–36.

    Zandi PP, Carlson MC, Plassman BL, et al. Hormone replacement therapy and incidence of Alzheimer disease in older women: The Cache County Study. JAMA. 2002;288:2123–29.

68. M. Fox, "Jellyfish Memory Supplement Prevagen Is a Hoax, FTC Says," NBC News, February 7, 2017; https://www.nbcnews.com/health/health-news/jellyfish-memory-supplement-prevagen-hoax-ftc-says-n704886.
69. Answer by Jonathan Graff-Radford at https://www.mayoclinic.org/diseases-conditions/alzheimers-disease/expert-answers/alzheimers-prevention/faq-20058140.
70. Melby-Lervåg M, Redick TS, Hulme C. Working memory training does not improve performance on measures of intelligence or other measures of 'far transfer': Evidence from a meta-analytic review. Perspec Psychol Sci. 2016;11:512–34.
71. Shipstead Z, Hicks KL, Engle RW. Cogmed working memory training: Does the evidence support the claims? J Appl Res Mem Cog. 2012;1:185–93.
72. Redick TS. Working memory training and interpreting interactions in intelligence interventions. Intelligence. 2015;50:14–20.
73. Simons DJ, Boot WR, Charness N, et al. Do "brain-training" programs work? Psychol Sci Public Interest 2016;17:103–86.
74. Nilsson J, Lebedev AV, Rydström A, Lövdén M. Direct-current stimulation does little to improve the outcome of working memory training in older adults. Psychol Sci. 2017;28:907–20.
75. http://www.telegraph.co.uk/news/health/news/10964854/One-hour-of-exercise-a-week-can-halve-dementia-risk.html.
76. Blondell SJ, Hammersley-Mather R, Veerman JL. Does physical activity prevent cognitive decline and dementia? A systematic review and meta-analysis of longitudinal studies. BMC Public Health. 2014;14:510.
77. Brasure M, Desai P, Davila H, et al. Physical activity interventions in preventing cognitive decline and Alzheimer-type dementia: A systematic review. Ann Intern Med. 2018;168:30–38.
78. S. Carpenter, "Does Estrogen Protect Memory?," *American Psychological Association Monitor* (January 2001): 52.

79. Shah S, Bell RJ, Davis SR. Homocysteine, estrogen and cognitive decline. Climacteric. 2006;9:77–87.

80. Henderson VW, Espeland MA, Hogan PE, et al. Prior use of hormone therapy and incident Alzheimer's disease in the Women's Health Initiative study. Neurol. 2007;68:8205.

Chapter 6: Can Breast Cancer Survivors Take Estrogen?

1. Bluming AZ, Dosik G, Lowitz B, Newman S, Citronbaum R, Zeitz B, Rosenbaum C, Rossman S, Drickman M, Sievers D, Marks R, Schlesinger M, Morrow D, Cowen S, Portnoff C, Harwood R, Koenig N, Green J, Calmenson M, Raphael H, Pomerantz A, Gittleman N, Kovner L, Kalan H, Baum R, Ozohan ML, Thompson R, Greenberg S, Fingerhut A, Frey H, Lewinsky B, Green N, Winkler L, Sillman H, Bricklin A, Garfinkle J, Bernstein D, Protzel R, Belzer J. Treatment of primary breast cancer without mastectomy: The Los Angeles community experience and review of the literature. Ann Surg. 1986;204:136–47.

2. Creasman WT. HRT and women who have had breast or endometrial cancer. J Epidemiol Biostat. 1999;4:217–25.

3. Gail MH, Benichou J. Assessing the risk of breast cancer in individuals. Cancer Prev. 1991;1:1–15.

4. MacMahon B, Cole P, Lin M, et al. Age at first birth and breast cancer risk. Bull WHO. 1970;43:209–21.

5. Lambertini M, Kroman N, Ameye L, et al. Long-term safety of pregnancy following breast cancer according to estrogen receptor status. J Natl Cancer Inst 2018; 110:426–9.

6. Wile AG, DiSaia PJ. Hormones and breast cancer. Am J Surg. 1989;157:438–42.

   DiSaia PJ, Brewster WR, Ziogas A, Anton-Culver H. Breast cancer survival and hormone replacement therapy: A cohort analysis. Am J Clin Oncol. 2000;23:541–45.

7. Huggins C, Moon RC, Morii S. Extinction of experimental mammary cancer. I. Estradiol-17beta and progesterone. PNAS. 1962;48:379–86.

8. Palshof T, Mouridsen HT, Daehnfeldt JL. Adjuvant endocrine therapy of primary operable breast cancer: Report on the Copenhagen breast cancer trials. Eur J Cancer. 1980;1:183–87.

   Palshof T, Carstensen B, Mouridsen HT, Dombernowsky P. Adjuvant endocrine therapy in pre- and postmenopausal women with operable breast cancer. Rev Endocrine Related Cancer. 1985; 17:43–50.

9. Beex L, Pieters PG, Smals A, et al. Tamoxifen versus ethinyl estradiol in the treatment of postmenopausal women with advanced breast cancer. Cancer Treat Rep. 1981;65:179–85.

10. Stoll BA. Effect of Lyndiol, an oral contraceptive, on breast cancer. BMJ. 1967;1:150–53.

11. Baum M. Hormone replacement therapy in breast cancer. Letter to the editor. Lancet. 1994;343:53.

12. Bluming AZ: Hormone replacement therapy: Benefits and risks for the general postmenopausal female population and for women with a history of previously-treated breast cancer. Semin Oncol. 1993;20:662–74.

13. Golden L, Stadel B. Estrogen replacement therapy in breast cancer survivors. Letter to the editor. JAMA. 1995;273:620–21.

14. Bluming AZ. Hormone replacement therapy (HRT) in women with previously treated primary breast cancer: Update XIV. Proc ASCO J Clin Oncol. 2008;15s:20693.

15. Cobleigh MA, Berris RF, Bush T, et al. Estrogen replacement therapy in breast cancer survivors: A time for change. Breast Cancer Committees of the Eastern Cooperative Oncology Group. JAMA. 1994;272:540–45.

16. Verheul HA, Coelingh-Bennick HJ, Kenemans P, et al. Effects of estrogens and hormone replacement therapy on breast cancer risk

and on efficacy of breast cancer therapies. Maturitas. 2000; 36:1–17.

17. Ylikorkala O, Metsä-Heikkilä M. Hormone replacement therapy in women with a history of breast cancer. Gynecol Endocrinol. 2002;16:469–78.

18. Uršič-Vrščaj M, Bebar S. A case-control study of hormone replacement therapy after primary surgical breast cancer treatment. Eur J Surg Oncol. 1999;25:146–51.

19. Eden JA, Bush T, Nand S, et al. A case-control study of combined continuous estrogen-progestin replacement therapy among women with a personal history of breast cancer. Menopause. 1995;2:67–72.

20. Dew J, Eden J, Beller E, et al. A cohort study of hormone replacement therapy given to women previously treated for breast cancer. Climacteric. 1998;1:137–42.

Dew JE, Wren BG, Eden JA. Tamoxifen, hormone receptors and hormone replacement therapy in women previously treated for breast cancer: A cohort study. Climacteric. 2002;5:151–55.

21. Durna EM, Wren BG, Heller GZ, et al. Hormone replacement therapy after a diagnosis of breast cancer: Cancer recurrence and mortality. Med J Aust. 2002;177:347–51.

Durna EM, Heller GZ, Leader LR, et al. Breast cancer in premenopausal women: Recurrence and survival rates and relationship to hormone replacement therapy. Climacteric. 2004;7: 284–91.

22. Espie M, Gorins A, Perret F, et al. Hormone replacement therapy (HRT) in patients treated for breast cancer: Analysis of a cohort of 120 patients. Proc ASCO. 1999(abstract);18:2262.

23. Marttunen MB, Hietanen P, Pyrhonen S, et al. A prospective study on women with a history of breast cancer and with or without estrogen replacement therapy. Maturitas. 2001;39:217–25.

24. Beckmann MW, Jap D, Djahansouzi S, et al. Hormone replacement therapy after treatment of breast cancer: Effects on postmeno-

pausal symptoms, bone mineral density and recurrence rates. Oncol. 2001;60:199–206.

25. Vassilopoulou-Sellin R, Asmar L, Hortobagyi GN, et al. Estrogen replacement therapy after localized breast cancer: Clinical outcome of 319 women followed prospectively. J Clin Oncol. 1999;17: 1482–87.

26. Brewster WR, DiSaia PJ, Grosen EA, et al. Experience with estrogen replacement therapy in breast cancer survivors. Int J Fertil Women's Med. 1999;44:186–92.

27. Decker DA, Pettinga JE, Vander Velde N, et al. Estrogen replacement therapy in breast cancer survivors: A matched-controlled series. Menopause. 2003;10:277–85.

28. Peters GN, Fodera T, Sabol J, et al. Estrogen replacement therapy after breast cancer: A 12-year follow-up. Ann Surg Oncol. 2001;8: 828–32.

29. O'Meara ES, Rossing MA, Daling JR, et al. Hormone replacement therapy after a diagnosis of breast cancer in relation to recurrence and mortality. J Natl Cancer Inst. 2001;93:754–62.

30. Meurer LN, Lená S. Cancer recurrence and mortality in women using hormone replacement therapy: Meta-analysis. J Fam Pract. 2002;51:1056–62.

31. Ettinger B, Grady D, Tosteson AN, et al. Effect of the Women's Health Initiative on women's decisions to discontinue postmenopausal hormone therapy. Obstet Gynecol. 2003;102:1225–32.

32. E-mail from Michelle Fujimoto to Avrum Bluming, December 20, 2017. Reprinted with her permission.

33. Letter from Dr. Philip DiSaia to Avrum Bluming, January 3, 2007. Quoted with his permission.

34. Chlebowski RT, Col N. Menopausal hormone therapy after breast cancer. Lancet. 2004;363:410–11.

35. Holmberg L, Anderson H. HABITS (hormonal replacement therapy after breast cancer—is it safe?). A randomized comparison: Trial stopped. Lancet. 2004;363:453–55.

36. Holmberg L, Iversen OE, Rudenstam CM, et al. Increased risk of recurrence after hormone replacement therapy in breast cancer survivors. J Natl Cancer Inst. 2008;100:475–82.

37. Von Schoultz E, Rutqvist LE. Menopausal hormone therapy after breast cancer: The Stockholm randomized trial. J Natl Cancer Inst. 2005;97:533–35.

    For the follow-up, see Fahlén M, Fornander T, Johansson H, et al. Hormone replacement therapy after breast cancer: 10 year follow-up of the Stockholm randomized trial. Eur J Cancer. 2013;49:52–59.

38. Creasman WT. Hormone replacement therapy after cancers. Curr Opin Oncol. 2005;17:496.

39. Ibid., 497.

40. Mueck AO, Rabe T, Kiesel L, Strowitzki T. Hormone replacement therapy after breast cancer. J Reprod Med Endocrinol. 2008;5:83.

41. Society of Obstetricians and Gynecologists of Canada (SOGC). Use of hormonal replacement therapy after treatment of breast cancer. Int J Gynecol Obstet. 2005;88:216–21.

42. Quoted in Zielinski SL. Hormone replacement therapy for breast cancer survivors: An answered question? J Natl Cancer Inst. 2005;97:955.

43. Holmberg L, Anderson H. Stopping HABITS. Lancet. 2004; 363:1477.

44. Batur P, Blixen CE, Moore HCF, et al. Menopausal hormone therapy (HT) in patients with breast cancer. Maturitas. 2006;53: 123–32.

45. Cobleigh MA, Berris RF, Bush T, et al. Estrogen replacement therapy in breast cancer survivors: A time for change. Breast Cancer Committees of the Eastern Cooperative Oncology Group. JAMA. 1994;272:540–45.

46. S. Mukherjee, The Laws of Medicine: Field Notes from an Uncertain Science (New York: Simon and Schuster, 2015), 4.

Chapter 7: Progesterone and the Pill

1. Stefanick ML, Anderson GL, Margolis KL, et al. for the WHI Investigators. Effects of conjugated equine estrogens on breast cancer and mammography screening in postmenopausal women with hysterectomy. JAMA. 2006;295:1647–57.

   For the WHI follow-up: Manson JE, Chlebowski RT, Stefanick ML, et al. Menopausal hormone therapy and health outcomes during the intervention and extended poststopping phases of the Women's Health Initiative Randomized Trials. JAMA. 2013;310:1352–68.

2. Roehm E. A reappraisal of Women's Health Initiative estrogen-alone trial: Long-term outcomes in women 50–59 years of age. Obstet Gynecol Int. 2015; article ID 713295, doi.org/10.1155/2015/713295.

3. Anderson GL, Limacher M, Assaf AR, et al. Effects of conjugated equine estrogen in postmenopausal women with hysterectomy: The Women's Health Initiative Randomized Controlled Trial. JAMA. 2004;291:1701–12.

   Viscoli CM, Brass LM, Kernan WN, et al. A clinical trial of estrogen replacement therapy after ischemic stroke. N Engl J Med. 2001;345:1243–49.

   Ross RK, Paganini-Hill A, Wan PC, et al. Effect of hormone replacement therapy on breast cancer risk: Estrogen versus estrogen plus progestin. J Natl Cancer Inst. 2000;92:328–32.

   Chen CL, Weiss NS, Newcomb P, et al. Hormone replacement therapy in relation to breast cancer. JAMA. 2002;287:734–41.

   Porch JV, Lee IM, Cook NR, et al. Estrogen-progestin replacement therapy and breast cancer risk: The Women's Health Study. Cancer Causes Control. 2002;13:847–54.

   Weiss LK, Burkman RT, Cushing-Haugen KL, et al. Hormone replacement therapy regimens and breast cancer risk. Obstet Gynecol. 2002;100:1148–58.

Li CI, Malone KE, Porter PL, et al. Relationship between long durations and different regimens of hormone therapy and risk of breast cancer. JAMA. 2003;289:3254–63.

Olsson HL, Ingvar C, Bladstrom A. Hormone replacement therapy containing progestogens and given continuously increases breast carcinoma risk in Sweden. Cancer. 2003;97:1387–92.

4. Van Veelen H, Willemse PHB, Tjabbes T, et al. Oral high-dose medroxyprogesterone acetate versus tamoxifen: A randomized crossover trial in postmenopausal patients with advanced breast cancer. Cancer. 1986;58:7–13.

See also Parazzini F, Colli E, Scatigna M, et al. Treatment with tamoxifen and progestins for metastatic breast cancer in postmenopausal women: A quantitative review of published randomized clinical trials. Oncol. 1993;50:483–89.

5. Badwe R, Hawlader R, Parmar V, et al. Single-injection depot progesterone before surgery and survival in women with operable breast cancer: A randomized controlled trial. J Clin Oncol. 2011;29:2845–51.

See also Badwe RA, Wang DY, Gregory WM, et al. Serum progesterone at the time of surgery and survival in women and premenopausal operable breast cancer. Eur J Cancer. 1994;30A:445–48.

6. Grattarola R. The premenstrual endometrial pattern of women with breast cancer: A study of pro-gestational activity. Cancer. 1964;17:1119–22.

Cowan LD, Gordis L, Tonascia JA, Jones GS. Breast cancer incidence in women with a history of progesterone deficiency. Am J Epidemiol. 1981;114:209–17.

7. Strom BL, Berlin JA, Weber AL, et al. Absence of an effect of injectable and implantable progestin-only contraceptives on subsequent risk of breast cancer. Contraception. 2004;69:353–60.

8. Mohammed H, Russell A, Stark R, et al. Progesterone receptor modulates estrogen receptor-α action in breast cancer. Nature. 2015;523:313–17.

Carroll JS, Hickey TE, Tarulli GA, et al. Deciphering the

divergent roles of progestogen in breast cancer. Nat Rev. Cancer. 2017;17:54–64.

9. Kuhl H, Stevenson J. The effect of medroxyprogesterone acetate on estrogen-dependent risks and benefits—an attempt to interpret the Women's Health Initiative results. Gynecol Endocrinol. 2006;22:303–17.

10. Santen RJ, Pinkerton J, McCartney C, et al. Risk of breast cancer with progestins in combination with estrogen as hormone replacement therapy. J Clin Endocrinol Metab. 2001;86:21.

11. Micheli A, Muti P, Secreto G, et al. Endogenous sex hormones and subsequent breast cancer in pre-menopausal women. Int J Cancer. 2004;112:312–18.

   Berrino F, Muti P, Micheli A, et al. Serum sex hormone levels after menopause and subsequent breast cancer. J Natl Cancer Inst. 1996;88:291–96.

12. Gadducci A, Biglia N, Cosio S, et al. Progestagen component and combined hormone replacement therapy in postmenopausal women and breast cancer risk: A debated clinical issue. Gynecol Endocrinol. 2009;25:807–15.

13. Campagnoli C, Abba C, Ambrogio S, et al. Pregnancy, progesterone and progestins in relation to breast cancer risk. J Steroid Biochem Mol Biol. 2005;97:441–50.

   Campagnoli C, Clavel-Chapelon F, Kaaks R, et al. Progestins and progesterone and hormone replacement therapy and the risk of breast cancer. J Steroid Biochem Mol Biol. 2005;96:95–108.

   Sitruk-Ware R. Progestogens in a hormonal replacement therapy: New molecules, risks, and benefits. Menopause. 2002;9:6–15.

   De Lignières B, de Vathaire F, Fournier S, et al. Combined hormone replacement therapy and risk of breast cancer in a French cohort study of 3175 women. Climacteric. 2002;5:332–40.

   Fournier A, Berrino F, Riboli E, et al. Breast cancer risk in relation to different types of hormone replacement therapy in the E3N-EPIC cohort. Int J Cancer. 2005;114:448–54.

Fournier A, Berrino F, Clavel-Chapelon F. Unequal risk for breast cancer associated with different hormone replacement therapies: Results from E3N cohort study. Breast Cancer Res Treat. 2008;107:103–11.

Murkes D, Conner P, Leifland K, et al. Effects of percutaneous estradiol-oral progesterone versus oral conjugated equine estrogens-medroxyprogesterone acetate on breast cell proliferation and Bcl-2 protein in healthy women. Fertil Steril. 2011;95:1188–91.

14. Siegel RL, Miller KD, Jemal A. Cancer statistics, 2018. CA: Cancer J Clin. 2018;68:7–30.

15. Barzi A, Lenz AM, Labonte MJ, et al. Molecular pathways: Estrogen pathway in colorectal cancer. Clin Cancer Res. 2013;19: 5842–48.

16. Hendifar A, Yang D, Lenz F, et al. Gender disparities in metastatic colorectal cancer survival. Clin Cancer Res. 2009;15:6391–97.

Fernandez E, Bosetti C, La Vecchia C, et al. Sex differences in colorectal cancer mortality in Europe, 1955–1996. Eur J Cancer Prev. 2000;9:99–104.

Hildebrand JS, Jacobs EJ, Campbell PT, et al. Colorectal cancer incidence and postmenopausal hormone use by type, recency, and duration in cancer prevention study II. Cancer Epidemiol Biomarkers Prev. 2009;18:2835–41.

Tannen RL, Weiner MG, Die D, et al. A simulation using data from a primary care practice database closely replicated the Women's Health Initiative trial. J Clin Epidemiol. 2007;60:686–95.

Rennert G, Rennert HS, Pinchev M, et al. Use of hormone replacement therapy and the risk of colorectal cancer. J Clin Oncol. 2009;27:4542–47.

Green J, Czanner G, Reeves G, et al. Menopausal hormone therapy and risk of gastrointestinal cancer: Nested case-control study within a prospective cohort, and meta-analysis. Int J Cancer. 2012;130:2387–96.

Calle EE, Miracle-McMahill HL, Thun MJ, et al. Estrogen replacement therapy and risk of fatal colon cancer in a prospective cohort of postmenopausal women. J Natl Cancer Inst. 1995;87: 517–23.

Slattery ML, Anderson K, Samovitz W, et al. Hormone replacement therapy and improved survival among postmenopausal women diagnosed with colon cancer (USA). Cancer Causes Control. 1999;10:467–73.

Mandelson MT, Miglioretti D, Newcomb PA, et al. Hormone replacement therapy in relation to survival in women diagnosed with colon cancer. Cancer Causes Control. 2003;14:979–84.

Chan JA, Meyerhardt JA, Chan AT, et al. Hormone replacement therapy and survival after colorectal cancer diagnosis. J Clin Oncol. 2006;24:5680–86.

17. Tsilidis KK, Allen NE, Key TJ, et al. Menopausal hormone therapy and risk of colorectal cancer in the European Prospective Investigation into Cancer and Nutrition. Int J Cancer. 2011;128: 1881–89.

Newcomb PA, Chia VM, Hampton JM, et al. Hormone therapy in relation to survival from large bowel cancer. Cancer Causes Control. 2009;20:409–16.

18. Hartz A, He T, Ross JJ. Risk factors for colon cancer and 150,912 postmenopausal women. Cancer Causes Control. 2012;23: 1599–605.

Hoffmeister M, Raum E, Krtschil A, et al. No evidence for variation in colorectal cancer risk associated with different types of postmenopausal hormone therapy. Clin Pharmacol Ther. 2009; 86:416–24.

19. Vessey MP, Doll R. Investigation of relation between use of oral contraceptives and thromboembolic disease. BMJ. 1968;2:199–205.

20. Kiley J, Hammond C. Combined oral contraceptives: A comprehensive review. Clin Obstet Gynecol. 2007;50:868–77.

21. Kaunitz AM. Clinical practice: Hormonal contraception in women of older reproductive age. N Engl J Med. 2008;358:1262.

Ratner S, Ofri D. Menopause and hormone-replacement therapy. Part 2. Hormone-replacement therapy regimens. West J Med. 2001;175(1):32–34.

22. Centers for Disease Control, Cancer and Steroid Hormone Study. Long-term oral contraceptive use and the risk of breast cancer. JAMA. 1983;249:1591–95.

Centers for Disease Control. Oral contraceptive (OC) use and the risk of breast cancer in young women. MMWR. 1984;33:353–54.

Cancer and Steroid Hormone (CASH) Study of the Centers for Disease Control and the National Institute of Child Health and Human Development. Oral-contraceptive use and the risk of breast cancer. N Engl J Med. 1986;315:405–11.

Murray P, Stadel BV, Schlesselman JJ. Oral contraceptive use in women with a family history of breast cancer. Obstet Gynecol. 1989;73:977–83.

23. Marchbanks PA, McDonald JA, Wilson HG, et al. Oral contraceptives and the risk of breast cancer. N Engl J Med. 2002;346:2025–32.

24. Hannaford PC, Selvaraj S, Elliott AM, et al. Cancer risk among users of oral contraceptives: Cohort data from the Royal College of General Practitioners Oral Contraception Study. BMJ. 2007;335:651–58.

25. Figueiredo JC, Bernstein L, Capanu M, et al. for the WECARE Study Group. Oral contraceptives, postmenopausal hormones, and risk of asynchronous bilateral breast cancer: The WECARE Study Group. J Clin Oncol. 2008;26:1411–18.

Figueiredo JC, Haile RW, Bernstein L, et al. Oral contraceptives and postmenopausal hormones and risk of contralateral breast cancer among BRCA1 and BRCA2 mutation carriers and non-carriers: The WECARE Study. Breast Cancer Res Treat. 2010;120:175–83.

26. Hunter DJ, Colditz GA, Hankinson SE, et al. Oral contraceptive use and breast cancer: A prospective study of young women. Cancer Epidemiol Biomarkers Prev. 2010;19:2496–502.

27. Moorman PG, Havrilesky LJ, Gierisch JM, et al. Oral contraceptives and risk of ovarian cancer and breast cancer among high-risk women: A systematic review and meta-analysis. J Clin Oncol. 2013;31:4188–98.

28. Vessey MP, Doll R, Jones K, et al. An epidemiological study of oral contraceptives and breast cancer. BMJ. 1979;175:1757–60.

    Spencer JD, Millis RR, Hayward JL. Contraceptive steroids and breast cancer. BMJ. 1978;1:1024–26.

    Matthews PN, Millis RR, Hayward JL. Breast cancer in women who have taken contraceptive steroids. BMJ. 1981;282:772–76.

29. Siegel RL, Miller KD, Jemal A. Cancer statistics, 2018. CA: Cancer J Clin. 2018;68:7–30.

30. Kiley J, Hammond C. Combined oral contraceptives: A comprehensive review. Clin Obstet Gynecol. 2007;50:868–77.

31. Vessey MP, Painter R. Endometrial and ovarian cancer and oral contraceptives—findings in a large cohort study. Br J Cancer. 1995;71:1340–42.

    Vessey M, Yeates D, Flynn S. Factors affecting mortality in a large cohort study with special reference to oral contraceptive use. Contraception. 2010;82:221–29.

    Bast RC, Brewer M, Zou C, et al. Prevention and early detection of ovarian cancer: Mission impossible? Recent Results Cancer Res. 2007;174:91–100.

    Walker GR, Schlesselman JJ, Ness RB. Family history of cancer, oral contraceptive use, and ovarian cancer risk. Obstet Gynecol. 2002;186:8–14.

32. Collaborative Group on Hormonal Factors in Breast Cancer. Breast cancer and hormonal contraceptives: Collaborative reanalysis of individual data on 53,297 women with breast cancer and 100,239 women without breast cancer from 54 epidemiological studies. Lancet. 1996;347:1713–27.

33. ESHRE Capri Workshop Group. Hormones and breast cancer. Hum Reprod Update. 2004;10:281–93.

34. R. C. Rabin, "Birth Control Pills Still Linked to Breast Cancer, Study Finds," *New York Times,* December 6, 2017.

35. Mørch LS, Skovlund CW, Hannaford PC, et al. Contemporary hormonal contraception and the risk of breast cancer. N Engl J Med. 2017;377:2228–39.

36. Hunter DJ. Oral contraceptives and the small increased risk of breast cancer. N Engl J Med. 2017;377:2276–77.

37. Michels KA, Pfeiffer RM, Brinton LA, et al. Modification of the associations between duration of oral contraceptive use and ovarian, endometrial, breast, and colorectal cancers. JAMA Oncol. 2018;4:516–21.

38. Stuenkel C. More evidence why the product labeling for low-dose vaginal estrogen should be changed? Menopause. 2018;25: 4–6.

39. Crandall C J, Hovey, KM, Andrews CA, et al. Breast cancer, endometrial cancer, and cardiovascular events in participants who used vaginal estrogen in the Women's Health Initiative Observational Study. Menopause. 2018;25:11–20.

Chapter 8: Debates, Decisions, and Final Lessons in the Case for HRT

1. S. Love, *Dr. Susan Love's Menopause and Hormone Book* (New York: Random House, 2003), 23.

2. Ravdin's argument may be found here: Ravdin PM, Cronin KA, Howlader N, et al. The decrease in breast cancer incidence in 2003 in the United States. N Engl J Med. 2007;356:1670–74. The authors wrote: "Discontinuation of hormone replacement therapy could have caused a decreased incidence of breast cancer by direct hormonal effects on the growth of occult breast cancers, a change that would have been expected to affect predominantly estrogen-receptor-positive tumors."

   Avrum's rebuttal evidence may be found here: Decline in breast cancer incidence—United States: 1999–2003. MMWR. 2007;56:

549–53. "Age-adjusted incidence rates for *invasive breast cancer* [the kind that takes years to develop] decreased each year during 1999–2003, with the greatest decrease, 6.1%, occurring from 2002 to 2003." Rates of in situ breast cancer decreased only 2.7 percent.

3. Ravdin PM, Cronin KA, Chlebowski RT. A decline in breast cancer incidence. N Engl J Med. 2007;357:513.

   Ravdin et al.'s comment was in response to Bluming AZ. Correspondence: A decline in breast-cancer incidence. Letter to the editor. N Engl J Med. 2007;357:509–13.

   And also in response to Zahl P-H, Mæhlen J. A decline in breast-cancer incidence. Letter to the editor. N Engl J Med. 2007;357:509–13. These two Norwegian researchers noted, "In contrast to the results reported by Ravdin et al., from 2002 to 2005, breast-cancer incidence rates were stable in Norway and Sweden, despite a sharp decline in the use of hormone-replacement therapy."

4. Powledge T. Easing hormone anxiety. Scientific American. 2007;297:32–34.

5. Anderson GL, Chlebowski RT, Aragaki AK, et al. Conjugated equine oestrogen and breast cancer incidence and mortality in postmenopausal women with hysterectomy: Extended follow-up of the Women's Health Initiative randomised placebo-controlled trial. Lancet Oncol. 2012;13:476–86.

6. Garnet Anderson, quoted in Carol Ostrom, "Estrogen-Only Pills Cut Breast-Cancer Risk for Some," *Seattle Times,* March 6, 2012; https://www.seattletimes.com/seattle-news/estrogen-only-pills-cut-breast-cancer-risk-for-some/.

7. C. Smyth, "Women Told Hormone Replacement Therapy Does Not Lead to Early Death," *Times* (UK), September 13, 2017; https://www.thetimes.co.uk/article/women-told-hrt-does-not-lead-to-early-death-ztk08tn7j?shareToken=ad8acbab104dce49546d8e90d85b7987.

8. Manson JE, Aragaki AK, Rossouw JE, et al. Menopausal hormone therapy and long-term all-cause and cause-specific mortality: The

Women's Health Initiative Randomized Trials. JAMA. 2017;318: 927–38.

9. S. Sloman and P. Fernbach, *The Knowledge Illusion: Why We Never Think Alone* (New York: Riverhead Books, 2017), 160.

10. D. Kahneman, *Thinking, Fast and Slow* (New York: Farrar, Straus and Giroux, 2011), 276.

11. C. Tavris and E. Aronson, *Mistakes Were Made (but Not by Me)*, rev. ed. (Boston: Houghton Mifflin Harcourt, 2015).

12. Tatsioni A, Siontis GCM, Ioannidis JPA. Partisan perspectives in the medical literature: A study of high frequency editorialists favoring hormone replacement therapy. J Gen Intern Med. 2010; doi:10.1007/s11606-010-1360-7.

13. Vera-Badillo FE, Shapiro R, Ocana A, et al. Bias in reporting of end points of efficacy and toxicity in randomized, clinical trials for women with breast cancer. Ann Oncol. 2013;24:1238–44.

14. US Preventive Services Task Force Recommendation Statement. Hormone therapy for the primary prevention of chronic conditions in postmenopausal women. JAMA. 2017;318:2224–33.

15. Grady D. Evidence for postmenopausal hormone therapy to prevent chronic conditions: Success, failure, and lessons learned. Editorial. JAMA Intern Med. December 12, 2017, doi:10.1001/jamainternmed.2017.7861.

16. Visvanathan K, Levit LA, Raghavan D, et al. Untapped potential of observational research to inform clinical decision making: American Society of Clinical Oncology research statement. J Clin Oncol. 2017;35:1845–54.

17. Frieden TR. Evidence for health decision making—beyond randomized, controlled trials. N Engl J Med. 2017;377:465–75.

18. Lobo RA. Hormone replacement therapy: Current thinking. Nat Rev Endocrinol. 2017;13:220–31.

19. Shapiro S, Farmer RDT, Mueck AO, et al. Does hormone replacement therapy cause breast cancer? An application of causal principles to three studies. Part 2. The Women's Health Initiative:

Estrogen plus progestogen. J Fam Plann Reprod Health Care. 2011;37:165–72.

20. The 2017 hormone therapy position statement of the North American Menopause Society. Menopause. 2017;24:728–53.

21. Erdem U, Ozdegirmenci O, Sobaci E, et al. Dry eye in postmenopausal women using hormone replacement therapy. Maturitas. 2007;56:257–62.

    Schaumberg DA, Buring JE, Sullivan DA, et al. Hormone replacement therapy and dry eye syndrome. JAMA. 2001;286:2114–19.

22. Edelson RN. Menstrual migraine and other hormonal aspects of migraine. Headache. 1985;25:376–79.

23. Lobo RA. Hormone replacement therapy: Current thinking. Nat Rev Endocrinol. 2017;13:220–31.

24. Panay N, Hamoda H, Arya R, et al. The 2013 British Menopause Society and Women's Health Concern recommendations on hormone replacement therapy. Menopause Int. 2013;19:59–68.

    Pitkin J. Should HRT be duration limited? Menopause Int. 2013; 19:167–74.

25. The 2017 hormone therapy position statement of the North American Menopause Society. Menopause. 2017;24:728–53.

26. Prague JK, Roberts RE, Comninos AN, et al. Neurokinin 3 receptor antagonism rapidly improves vasomotor symptoms with sustained duration of action. Menopause. 2018;25:1–8.

27. Santen RJ, Allred DC, Ardoin SP, et al. Postmenopausal hormone therapy: An Endocrine Society scientific statement. J Clin Endocrinol Metab. 2010;95:S1–S66.

28. Zhao J-G, Zeng X-T, Wang J, Liu L. Association between calcium or vitamin D supplementation and fracture incidence in community-dwelling older adults: A systematic review and meta-analysis. JAMA. 2017;318:2466–82.

29. Santoro N, Braunstein GD, Butts CL. Compounded bioidentical hormones in endocrinology practice: An Endocrine Society scientific statement. J Clin Endocrinol Metab. 2016;101:1318–43.

30. Bhavnani BR, Strickler RC. Menopausal hormone therapy. J Ob-Gyn Canada 2005;27:137–62.

Shah S, Bell RJ, Davis SR. Homocysteine, estrogen and cognitive decline. Climacteric. 2006;9:77–87.

31. Brinton RD, Proffitt P, Tran J, Luu R. Equilin, a principal component of the estrogen replacement therapy Premarin, increases the growth of cortical neurons via an NMDA receptor-dependent mechanism. Exp Neurol. 1997;147:211–20.

32. Pickering G. Physician and scientist. Br. Med J. 1964,2:1615–9.

33. Blakemore C, Cooper GF. Development of the brain depends on the visual environment. Nature. 1970;228:477–78.

Afterword

1. Shifren JL, Crandall CJ, Manson JE. Menopausal hormone therapy. JAMA 2019;321:2458-9.

2. Chlebowski RT, Anderson GL, Aragaki AK. Association of menopausal hormone therapy with breast cancer incidence and mortality during long-term follow-up of the Women's Health Initiative Randomized Clinical Trials. JAMA 2020;324:369-80.

3. Hodis HN, Sarrel PM. Menopausal hormone therapy and breast cancer: what is the evidence from randomized trials? Climacteric 2018;21:521-8.

4. Chlebowski RT, Aragaki AK, Pan K. Breast cancer prevention: Time for change. J Clin Oncol Prac 2021 doi: 10.1200/OP.21.00343. Online ahead of print.

5. Lambertini M, Kroman N, Ameye L. Long-term safety of pregnancy following breast cancer according to estrogen receptor status. J Natl Cancer Inst 2018;110:426-9.

Lambertini M, Ameye L, Hamy A-S, et al. Pregnancy after breast cancer in patients with germline BRCA mutations. J Clin Oncol 2020;38:3012-23.

6. https://peterattiamd.com/hormone-therapy-and-breast-cancer/.

Index

Note: Italic page numbers refer to tables.

Adami, Hans-Olov, 24–25
Albright, Fuller, 110–11
Alzheimer's disease: alternative treatments for, 153–54, 236–37; anatomical aberrations in brains of patients, 137–38; estrogen's role in decreasing risk of, 130, 137, 139–40, 145–46, 151–52, 159–60, 236; gene variant for, 127–28; and HRT, 6, 7, 146, 237; prevention of, 129–30, 154; studies on prevention of, 139–40, 145–46; women's risk for, 7, 127, 129, 236
American Cancer Society, 7, 22, 83, 166
American College of Obstetrics and Gynecology, 69, 78
American Heart Association, 84, 85, 88
American Society of Clinical Oncology, 178–80, 225
Anderson, Garnet, 28–29, 147–48, 217, 218
androgen receptors, 199–200, 204
antidepressants, 70–71, 75–76, 78, 232
antiseizure medication, 75, 232
anxiety attacks, 5, 56, 59
APOE4, 127–28, 135, 145
atherosclerosis, 94–97, 103, 149, 160–61, 231

Badwe, Rajendra, 197–98
Barrett-Connor, Elizabeth, 25, 89
Baum, Michael, 71, 172
Beex, Louk V. A. M., 171–72

Bergkvist, Leif, 24–25
bioidentical products, 60, 74, 78–81, 235–36
birth control pills, 195, 201–8
bisphosphonates, 116, 119–21, 125, 191, 228, 234, 235
blood clots, 74, 114, 202, 223–24, 231
Boardman, Henry, 149–50
bone health: alternative treatments for, 114–23, 234–35; and balance between growth and loss, 106–7, 118; bone density versus bone resilience, 109–14, 116–17, 121–22, 125; and fractures, 105–7, 120; and fragility, 106, 117, 120; and HRT, 15, 124, 218, 231. *See also* hip fractures; osteoporosis
bone mineral density (BMD) tests, 115, 117–19
botanicals and natural products, 74, 76–78, 80
brain: anatomical and neurological changes in, 136, 138–39; blood-flow patterns, 140–42, 160; and estrogen's protective effects, 135, 140–42, 150–53, 161; and glial cells, 136–37, 137n, 138; neuroplasticity of, 137, 139, 142; transcranial direct-current stimulation for, 156–57
brain neurons, 136–40, 137n, 160, 236
BRCA gene, 23–24, 87, 204, 217

breast cancer: and biopsies for benign breast disease, 21; and birth control pills, 195, 201–8; cure rate for, 5, 53, 83, 175, 240; diagnosis of, 3–4, 11–12, 182, 204–5; family history of, 22, 102, 149, 203, 209, 217; fears of, 8, 9, 15–16, 53, 84, 109, 114, 128, 179n, 240; fund-raising efforts for, 85, 87; history of treatment of, 9, 18; invasive breast cancers, 26, 29, 52, 161, 192, 197, 198, 206, 215; localized breast cancer, 53; and lymph-node involvement, 188, 189, 198; noninvasive breast cancer, 52, 215; risk statistics on, 4–5, 10–11, 13, 23, 36, 37–38, 49, 83, 102, 170, 218, 221, 224; role of hormones in cause of, 9, 10–12, 13, 20, 24, 25–26, 34–35, 42–46, 53, 54, 83, 96, 114, 169, 224; treatment with estrogen, 50–51; women's risk for Alzheimer's compared to, 129; women's risk for heart disease compared to, 83–84, 84, 85, 86, 87–88, 234, 240

breast cancer survivors: and birth control pills, 203, 204; and HRT, 6, 15, 72, 163, 168, 169–76, 194, 237; and onset of menopause from chemotherapy, 71–72; pilot study on effects of HRT for, 176–81; premenopausal women as, 169–71; proposal of pilot study on effects of HRT for, 173–76; SERMS given to postmenopausal survivors, 88, 121; studies on effects HRT for, 181–85, 187–90, 191, 192, 193

Brewster, Wendy, 183–84

Brinton, Roberta Diaz, 134, 139–40, 150–51, 236

British Menopause Society and Women's Health Concern, 231–32

Brownstein, David, 78–79

calcium supplements, 75, 105, 110–12, 116–17, 125, 228, 234–35

cancer: women's risk for, 84, 93, 218–19. See also specific types of cancer

Cancer Journal, 13, 220

Carroll, Jason, 198–99

CASH Study, 203

causation: chain of evidence for, 43, 44; and correlation, 44–46, 47, 49; and Hill criteria, 46–52, 53; and Koch's postulates, 42–43, 44, 45; and mosaic of evidence, 45, 46, 48, 51, 205, 225

Centers for Disease Control, 203, 207, 209

chemotherapy, 5, 66–67, 71–72

Chlebowski, Rowan, 187, 191

Climacteric, 13, 220, 241

Cobleigh, Melody, 179–80, 193

Cochrane analysis, 149–50, 225

cognitive functioning: effects of estrogen on, 142, 143–45, 151–52, 159–60, 161; and exercise, 154, 157–59, 228; and transcranial direct-current stimulation, 156–57

cognitive impairment: and aging, 128, 131; and ERT, 133–34, 135, 136, 151–52, 160; and HRT, 67, 131, 133–34, 135, 146, 152, 233; measurement of, 158. See also stroke

Col, Nananda, 22, 102, 113

Collaborative Group on Hormonal Factors in Breast Cancer, 205–6, 207

Collaborative Reanalysis, 25–26

colon cancer, 6–7, 201, 207, 209, 224

Creasman, William, 169–70, 189–90, 191

data mining, 36, 38–41, 52, 220, 227

Dean, Cornelia, 94–95

dementia: causes of, 116; and ERT, 132–35, 137, 151; fears of, 128; and HRT, 130–34, 135, 146, 151, 162, 180, 224; and physical activity, 157, 158–59, 236–37. See also Alzheimer's disease

dendrites, 138, 140

depression, 56–59, 70–71, 172

Dew, Jennifer, 181–82

diabetes, 84, 218, 224

diethylstilbestrol (DES), 51, 171

DiSaia, Philip, 170, 183–84, 186–87, 191
dual-energy X-ray absorptiometry (DXA),
    117, 119

endometrial cancer, 5–6, 11, 19, 114, 207,
    208, 218
Engel, Randall W., 155–56
epidemiological studies, 35–36, 44–48, 89,
    205–6
ERA study, 95
estradiol, 79, 79n, 171, 235
estrogen: benefits for the brain, 135,
    140–42, 150–53, 161; cardiovascular
    benefits of, 89, 93; Hill criteria applied
    to, 49–51; and hypothesis of cause of
    breast cancer, 9, 10–12, 13, 24, 25–26,
    34–35, 42–46, 53, 54, 83, 96, 114,
    213–14, 221; marketing of, 64–65; in
    patch form, 201, 236; and risk of
    Alzheimer's disease, 130, 137, 139, 140,
    145–46, 151, 152, 159, 160, 236; and risk
    of recurrence of breast cancer, 72,
    170–71; risks of, 15, 21, 72–73, 101, 195,
    212–13; side effects of, 98; therapeutic
    benefits of, 15, 62, 101–2; as treatment
    for metastatic breast cancer, 10, 51;
    women's cumulative levels of, 10–11,
    40–41, 50, 221. See also Premarin
Estrogen Prevention of Atherosclerosis Trial
    (EPAT), 95
estrogen replacement therapy (ERT):
    benefits of, 15, 223; and brain's
    neuroplasticity, 137; and cognitive
    functioning, 143–44; and cognitive
    impairment, 133–34, 135, 136, 151–52,
    160; and dementia, 132–35, 137, 151;
    endometrial cancer associated with, 5–6,
    19; and heart disease, 93, 95–96, 102–3,
    218; history of, 18–19, 60–65; and
    menopausal symptoms, 69, 102–3, 227;
    and pharmaceutical industry, 123–24;
    for prevention of hip fractures, 6,
    112–14, 121, 124–25, 234, 235; and

prognosis for breast cancer diagnosis, 10;
    risks of, 15, 41, 223–24; studies of,
    20–21, 22, 23, 24–25, 34–35, 40, 41, 49,
    50, 54, 70, 152; as term, 6n; Women's
    Health Initiative on, 23, 73, 196–97, 227
Ettinger, Bruce, 114, 116, 118
evidence: chain of, 43, 44; and clinical
    judgment, 165; evidence-based medical
    care, 91; interpretation of, 220; mosaic
    of, 45, 46, 48, 51, 205, 225
Ewing's sarcoma, 167–68, 169
exercise: for bone health, 116–17, 125; for
    cognitive functioning, 154, 157–59, 228;
    and dementia, 157, 158–59, 236–37;
    posture exercise, 107

feminism, 60, 61–62, 81, 220
Feynman, Richard, 17–18
Figueiredo, Jane, 203–4
Food and Drug Administration (FDA):
    on Alzheimer's medications, 130, 153;
    on bioidentical estrogen, 79, 235;
    black-box warnings of, 185–86, 210;
    on HRT for breast cancer survivors,
    173–76, 177, 179, 181, 187; on
    medications for hot flashes, 76; on
    osteoporosis medications, 123
Fosamax, 120, 122–23
Framingham Heart Study, 6, 99, 112

gabapentin (Neurontin), 75, 76, 232
gallbladder disease, 74, 224, 231
gender differences, 85, 86, 98, 99, 106, 129
glial cells, 136–37, 137n, 138, 140
Gorsky, Robin, 101–2
Grady, Deborah, 76–77, 113–14, 116, 224
Grob, Gerald N., 115–16, 118, 125

HABITS study, 187–91, 192
Hartz, Arthur, 91, 201
Healy, Bernadine, 7–8, 240
heart disease: and aspirin, 101, 191; and
    estrogen's cardiovascular benefits, 62, 89,

heart disease *(cont.)*
91, 160; HRT's effects on, 6, 7, 15, 62, 67, 82, 88–97, 101, 102–3, 149, 150, 180, 218, 227, 234; and statins, 83, 97–99, 101; strategies for reducing women's risk of, 97–100, 191; studies of women with preexisting heart disease, 147, 149; women's risk for, 7, 83–86, 217, 240; women's risk for breast cancer compared to, 83–84, *84*, 85, 86, 87–88, 234, 240

Higgins, Gus, 167–68

Hill, Austin Bradford, 46–52, 53, 92, 149–50

hip fractures: and calcium supplements, 111–12; and ERT, 6, 112–14, 124–25, 234, 235; and femurs, 105, 107, 120; and HRT, 112–13, 116, 119, 124; and length of HRT, 113–14, 234; medications reducing risk of, 121–23; and risk of death, 108–9, 234; and risk of falls, 106, 119

Holmberg, Lars, 187–88, 191

Holtorf, Kent, 78–79

Holtzman, David, 128, 129

Hoover, Robert, 53–54

hormone replacement therapy (HRT): benefits of, 6–8, 15, 21, 28, 33, 81–82, 194, 195, 200–201, 211, 219–20, 224, 242; and breast cancer survivors, 6, 15, 72, 163, 168, 169–76, 194, 237; and cognitive biases in research, 12; and dementia, 130–34, 135, 146, 151, 162, 180, 224; discontinuing of, 96–97, 152; effects on cognitive impairment, 67, 131, 133–34, 135, 146, 152, 233; effects on colon cancer, 201; effects on heart disease, 6, 7, 15, 62, 67, 82, 88–97, 101, 102–3, 149, 150, 180, 218, 227, 234; effects on menopausal symptoms, 15, 28, 57, 58, 67–69, 73, 82, 102–3, 113, 223, 230, 233–34, 242; history of, 60–65; individualization of, 69, 149, 240; and life expectancy, 7, 8, 22, 41, 101, 102, 103, 201, 209, 218, 225, 231, 237; litigation on,
186; and "lowest dose for shortest time" concept, 72–73, 232–33; Million Women Study on, 34–35; and pharmaceutical industry, 123–24; physicians' resistance to, 14–15; for prevention of hip fractures, 112–13, 116, 119, 124; and risk of Alzheimer's disease, 146, 151, 162; and risk of stroke, 147, 148, 149–50, 160, 218, 224, 228; risks of, 8, 13, 15, 21, 33, 41, 82, 194, 211, 215, 219–20, 224, 230–32, 242; side effects of, 74, 120, 224, 231, 242; studies of, 20–22, 23, 24–30, 36, 40–41, 49, 50–54, 69–71, 96, 222, 225; as term, 6n, 60–61; timing of, 101, 150–53, 160, 161, 162, 218, 230–31; Women's Health Initiative on, 26–33, 36, 51, 59, 66–68, 74, 78, 82, 132, 161–62, 196–97, 199, 214, 215, 216, 226, 227, 241–42

hot flashes: and birth control pills, 202; ERT for, 77; medications for, 75, 232; as symptom of menopause, 5, 56, 64, 66–67, 69, 72–73, 233

H. pylori, 43–44

hysterectomies, 19, 93, 144

Isoflavone Clover Extract Study, 76

IUDs, 206–7

Journal of the American Medical Association (JAMA): on birth control pills, 208; on calcium supplements, 111; on clinical trials for HRT, 176; on ERT, 41; on HRT, 7, 223; on idalopirdine, 130; on therapies for hot flashes, 77; and Women's Health Initiative, 26–27, 32, 33, 217, 218, 226

Kahneman, Daniel, 222, 238

Kennedy, Pagan, 127–28

Klingberg, Torkel, 154–55

Koch, Robert, 42–43, 44, 45

Kolata, Gina, 19, 62

Kotsopoulos, Joanne, 23–24

Lancet, 25–26, 34–35, 39, 84
Langer, Robert, 31–32, 121
Legato, Marianne, 85–86
Lená, Sarah, 184–85
life expectancy: and HRT, 7, 8, 22, 41, 102–3, 201, 209, 218, 225, 231, 237; of modern women, 66, 129
Lobo, Roger, 225–26, 231
Loh, Sandra Tsing, 58–59
Love, Susan, 211–13, 220
lumpectomy, 5, 9, 161, 165–67, 179, 192
lung cancer, 30, 36, *38,* 48–49, 51, 53, 83, 163–64

Maclaran, Kate, 147–48
Maki, Pauline, 134, 141, 152
Manson, JoAnn, 73–74, 82, 217, 218–19
Marshall, Barry, 43–44
mastectomy, 9–10, 13, 54, 165–66, 168–69, 179n. *See also* lumpectomy
Mastorakos, George, 148–49
Mayo Clinic, 51, 69, 114, 154, 157
medicine and medical care: causation in, 42–46; evidence-based, 91; feminist critique of, 81; paternalism of, 61, 65; physicians, 14–15, 33–34, 40, 46–52. *See also* scientific research
medroxyprogesterone acetate (MPA), 196, 197, 208
memory: benefits of estrogen for, 139, 141, 142, 143–45, 152–53; and brain pathology, 137–38; and glial cells, 136–37; memory loss, 63, 128; studies on, 130–35, 152–53; and Women's Health Initiative, 130–31, 134; working-memory training, 154–56, 157, 228
men, 85, 106, 110, 128–29, 146
menarche, early, 10–11, 50, 221
menopausal symptoms: and breast cancer survivors, 168, 169, 170, 172, 177–78, 180, 190, 193–94; effects of ERT on, 69, 102–3, 227; effects of HRT on, 15, 28, 57, 58, 67–69, 73, 82, 102–3, 113, 223,

230, 233–34, 242; lifestyle modifications for, 74–75; Premarin as treatment for, 19; severity of, 64, 66, 67, 68, 233; studies of, 177–78; types of, 5, 55–59, 63, 232; Women's Health Initiative on, 66–69, 70
menopause: alternative treatment of, 80, 80n; characterizations of, 64–66, 115, 212–13, 220; chemotherapy causing onset of, 5, 66–67, 71–72; definition of, 102; early menopause, 106, 116; and heart disease risk, 88–89; late menopause, 10–11, 50, 221
Metsä-Heikkilä, Merja, 180–81
Meurer, Linda N., 184–85
Mikkola, Tomi, 96–97
Million Women Study, 34–35, 40, 50

Nachtigall, Lila, 20, 62–63
National Cancer Institute, 20, 41, 53, 178–79, 192
National Institutes of Health (NIH), 7, 9, 26, 31–32, 112, 242
nerve growth factor (NGF), 140, 160
neurotransmitters, 138, 142
Neves-e-Castro, Manuel, 241–42
New England Journal of Medicine (NEJM), 6, 21–22, 24–25, 89, 91, 122, 206–7, 225
New York Times, 19, 62, 127, 129, 206–8, 209
night sweats, 56, 67, 69, 72–73, 233
North American Menopause Society, 27, 69, 73, 228–30, 232–33
Nurses' Health Study, 22, 40, 50, 89, 93, 96, 204

observational studies: on Alzheimer's disease, 145; on effects of HRT on breast cancer survivors, 190; methodological improvements in, 91; randomized controlled trials compared to, 27n, 90–92, 93, 100–101, 146–47, 224–25; and scientific research, 9, 27n, 90

osteoarthritis of the jaw, 70, 125, 235
osteopenia, 64, 118–20
osteoporosis: development of, 106–7, 120, 124; estrogen treatment for prevention of, 110, 112–13, 124–25; and HRT, 6, 7, 15, 62, 124–25, 149, 224, 228, 233; intervention versus diagnostic thresholds for, 118; medical diagnosis and treatment of, 115–23, 125; and osteomalacia, 110, 111; preventive treatment of, 119–20, 191, 228; and vertebrae, 107, 112, 114–15, 121, 123, 235; women's risk for, 7, 105–6, 119, 124, 125, 240
Our Bodies, Ourselves, 61
ovarian cancer, 23–24, 204–5, 207, 208
ovaries, 18, 89, 139, 143–44, 169–71

painful sexual intercourse, 5, 56, 63, 72, 232
palpitations, 5, 55–56, 57, 102, 232, 233, 234
parathyroid hormones, 121–22
Parker-Pope, Tara, 29, 32, 59
Patnaik, Jennifer, 87–88
Pearson, Cynthia, 62, 63–64
peptic ulcers, 43–44, 54
perimenopause, 57, 66, 202, 233
PET scans, 141, 141n
pharmaceutical industry, 14, 61, 64, 115–24, 210, 222
Pickering, George White, 237–38
Pike, Malcolm, 213–14, 215, 216
Postmenopausal Estrogen/Progestin Interventions trial (PEPI), 89
postmenopausal women: and breast cancer risk, 21, 23, 49, 213; and effect of estrogen on Alzheimer's disease risk, 130, 152; and effects of ERT, 23, 25, 89; and effects of estrogen on heart disease, 93; and effects of estrogen on hip fractures, 112, 113, 121; and effects of estrogen on memory, 145; and effects of HRT, 7, 20–21, 22, 102, 228; ERT for breast

cancer survivors, 170, 171–72; estrogen levels of, 137, 213; and exercise as treatment for bone health, 117, 125; hip fractures of, 108–9; HRT for breast cancer survivors, 172; HRT for prevention of chronic conditions in, 223; osteoporosis of, 110–12, 122–23; risk of stroke for, 146, 147; SERMs given to breast cancer survivors, 88; in Women's Health Initiative, 30, 67–68, 93–94, 95, 131, 220, 226
Pott, Percivall, 45–46
pregnancy, 11–12, 170, 171, 196
Premarin: forms of estrogen in, 79; production of, 18–19; risks of, 13; studies of, 20, 124, 143, 183, 188–89, 197, 235
premenopausal women, 117, 125, 137, 144–46, 182, 201
Prempro, 185–86, 196, 217
progesterone: in birth control pills, 202; bone formation stimulated by, 112; compounded bioidentical hormones as alternative to, 79; and HRT, 7, 19, 21–22, 24, 28, 172, 208–9; levels during pregnancy, 170, 196; micronized progesterone, 196, 200, 208, 209, 237; and risk of breast cancer, 171, 172, 195, 196–201; studies of, 197–99; synthetic forms of, 19, 196–200, 201, 204, 207–9, 237
progesterone-receptor-positive cells, 11, 199
Prometrium, 196, 208
Prospective Epidemiological Risk Factors Study, 146
Prospective Urban Rural Epidemiology (PURE) project, 99–100
Provera, 196, 200, 208

quality of life, 6, 8, 66–68, 72, 82, 160, 228, 230, 233–34

Rabin, Roni Caryn, 207–8
radical mastectomy, 9, 13, 54, 165, 168–69

raloxifene (Evista), 121, 235
randomized controlled trials (RCTs): and benefits of estrogen for female Alzheimer's patients, 151; on HRT for breast cancer survivors, 174, 175, 181, 187–89, 190, 191; observational studies compared to, 27n, 90–92, 93, 100–101, 146–47, 224–25; and participants' knowledge of placebos, 177–78; on removal of ovaries in premenopausal breast cancer survivors, 169–70; and scientific research, 9, 27, 27n, 29, 46, 68, 69–70, 90; of Women's Health Initiative, 27, 29, 68, 91, 150, 177, 220, 222
Ravdin, Peter, 214–16
Redick, Thomas S., 155, 156
Reitz, Rosetta, 61–62
REMEMBER study, 152–53
risk: absolute risks, 35–36, 41; relative risks, 35–36, *37–38*, 41. *See also specific diseases*
Rossouw, Jacques, 32–33, 92, 93, 97, 216, 219, 228

San Antonio Breast Cancer Symposium, 88, 191–92, 214–15
Schwartz, Erika, 78–79
scientific method, 48, 49, 52, 53–54
scientific research: advances in, 17–18; and advancing knowledge, 52; bias in, 222–23; causation in, 42–46; cognitive biases in, 12; and contextual and cultural factors, 219–20; conventions of, 32–34, 221, 237–38; and data mining, 35, 38–39, 52, 220, 227; and medical practice, 237–40; and observational studies, 9, 27n, 90; and randomized controlled trials, 9, 27, 27n, 29, 46, 68, 69–70, 90; and retrospective substratification, 38–41, 52; and statistical manipulation, 35–38; and theory-induced blindness, 222, 238–39
Seaman, Barbara, 61–62
Seaman, Gideon, 61–62

SERMs (selective estrogen-receptor modulators), 88, 121
sexual desire, loss of, 5, 19, 56, 59, 63, 69, 72
Sherwin, Barbara, 134, 143, 144, 151–52, 159–60
sleep problems, 5, 56–57, 67, 69–70, 72, 75, 102, 232–33
Speroff, Leon, 92, 134
spinal column, 107, 112, 114–15, 121, 123, 235
statins, 83, 97–99, 101, 191, 228, 234
Stefanick, Marcia, 216–17
Stockholm study, 189
stress, 42, 43, 54
stroke: and fat intake, 100; and HRT, 147, 148, 149–50, 160, 218, 224, 228; women's risk for, 7, 84, 85, 93, 146–50, 160–61, 217, 228
Study of Women's Health Across the Nation (SWAN), 66, 73

tamoxifen, 51, 171–72, 188–89, 190, 197, 221
Taubes, Gary, 44, 99
tau protein, 138, 140, 160
Taylor, Katie, 70–71, 81
theory-induced blindness, 222, 238–39
thyroid hormones, 60, 121
tobacco smoking, 36, *38*, 41, 48–49, 51, 53, 132, 226, 238
topical estrogen creams, 210, 232
transcranial direct-current stimulation (tDCS), 156–57
tuberculosis, 42, 54

U.S. Preventive Services Task Force (USPSTF), 223–24, 231
University of Wisconsin study, 6–7
urinary incontinence, 223, 224
urogenital atrophy, 63, 232
uterine cancer, 19–20
uterus, 143, 144–45

vaccinations, 44–45
vaginal discharge, 56, 69, 74
vaginal dryness, 5, 56, 69, 71, 232
vasomotor symptoms, 66, 69, 73, 202, 228
venous thrombosis, 93, 149, 231
vitamin D, 75, 110, 111, 210, 234–35

Warren, Robin, 43–44
Watkins, Elizabeth Siegel, 60, 61, 62, 69
WECARE study, 203–4
Wile, Alan, 170, 174
Wiley Protocol, 80–81
Wilson, Robert, 19, 64–65, 240
WISDOM study, 69–70
women: African American women, 66, 215; heart disease risk compared to breast cancer risk, 83–84, *84*, 85, 86, 87–88, 234, 240; life expectancy of, 66, 129. *See also* postmenopausal women; premenopausal women
Women's Health Initiative (WHI): on benefits of estrogen for prevention of hip fractures, 112–13; on bisphosphonates for risk of fractures, 120; on calcium and vitamin D supplements, 112; campaign of fear, 29–30, 33, 74, 114, 135, 219; claims concerning breast cancer, 28–29, 30, 36, 62, 96, 148, 185, 186–87, 191–92, 216, 226, 227, 228; Clinical Coordinating Center, 28–29; on colon cancer, 201; critical reassessment of methods, 30–32, 80, 93–95, 121, 134, 147–49, 217–18, 220, 226; data

manipulations of, 13, 31–34, 135, 148, 219, 227; on decline in breast cancer rates, 51; on dementia risk, 160; early termination of, 26–28, 29, 31–32, 33, 131, 134, 147, 148, 216, 226; on ERT, 23, 73, 196–97, 227; findings of, 8–9, 28, 31, 78, 101, 210, 211, 213, 216–19, 224, 225–26, 227; and global assessments, 68; health of women in sample, 30, 94, 132–33, 220, 226; and Hill criteria, 49; on HRT, 26–33, 36, 51, 59, 66–68, 74, 78, 82, 132, 161–62, 196–97, 199, 214, 215, 216, 226, 227, 241–42; on HRT's effect on heart disease, 92–94, 95, 227; influence of, 103, 185, 186–87, 191, 192, 214, 215; key problems with, 223–28; median age of women in sample, 30, 67, 94, 95, 226; on menopausal symptoms, 66–69, 70; on preventive treatment of osteoporosis, 119–20; on progesterone, 197, 199; randomized controlled trials of, 27, 29, 68, 91, 150, 177, 220, 222; representation of postmenopausal women in studies, 30, 67–68, 93–94, 95, 131, 220, 226; on risk of Alzheimer's disease, 152; statistical errors of, 35, 131–35, 226; on stroke risks, 147–48, 160–61, 217, 228
Women's Health Initiative Memory Study (WHIMS), 130–35
World Health Organization, 118, 119, 170
Wyeth, 14, 124, 185, 186

Ylikorkala, Olavi, 180–81

About the Authors

Avrum Bluming received his MD from the Columbia College of Physicians and Surgeons. He spent four years as a senior investigator for the National Cancer Institute and for two of those years was director of the Lymphoma Treatment Center in Kampala, Uganda. He organized the first study of lumpectomy for the treatment of breast cancer in Southern California in 1978, and for more than two decades he has been studying the benefits and risks of hormone replacement therapy administered to women with a history of breast cancer. Dr. Bluming has served as a clinical professor of medicine at USC and has been an invited speaker at the Royal College of Physicians in London and the Pasteur Institute in Paris. He was elected to mastership in the American College of Physicians, an honor accorded to only five hundred of the over one hundred thousand board-certified internists in this country.

Carol Tavris received her PhD in social psychology from the University of Michigan. Her books include *Mistakes Were Made (but Not by Me),* with Elliot Aronson; *Anger: The Misunderstood Emotion;* and *The Mismeasure of Woman.* She has written articles, op-eds, and book reviews on topics in psychological science for a wide array of publications—including the *Los Angeles Times,* the *New York Times Book Review,* the *Wall Street Journal,* and the *TLS*—and a column, "The Gadfly," for *Skeptic* magazine. She is a fellow of the Association for Psychological Science and has received numerous awards for her efforts to promote gender equality, science, and skepticism.